Elizabeth Prosser

A to Z of
Health, Sickness
and First Aid

ROBIN CLARK

First published in Great Britain 1976
by Barrie & Jenkins Ltd.
This edition published 1978 by Robin
Clark Ltd., 15 Leyden Road, Stevenage,
Herts, SG1 2BW

© Barrie & Jenkins Ltd 1976

Made and printed in Great Britain by
M C Print Co. Ltd., Stevenage, Herts.
ISBN 0 86072 012 8

CONTENTS

GOOD HEALTH

Good health is observable in the man or woman who has a sparkle in the eyes, a spring in the step, who eats and sleeps well, is wide-awake during the day, isn't overweight, and has a happy outlook on life.

Good health is an attitude of mind as well as a manner of living. If you do not live a healthy life, then all the medicines in the world won't put you right.

Live as close as you can to the way nature intended — get plenty of fresh air, exercise, keep clean, eat the right food, drink more water and less alcohol, avoid smoking, don't join the growing population of pill-takers, make the correct use of your sleep, and in this age of high-pressure living, never worry.

Cleanliness is essential, inside and out. Soap and water have no substitute. But much more important, internal cleanliness, through complete elimination of waste products, avoids that most chronic complaint, constipation. Don't overeat. Vary your diet, with lots of meat, fish, eggs, fresh fruit, green vegetables, salads, butter, wholemeal bread, cereals and milk to supply the necessary protein, carbo-hydrates, fat, vitamins and essential minerals.

Remember, being fat causes more diseases than not eating enough. And get plenty of fresh air and exercise at all ages.

Too many people hover between good health and poor health. This state can rarely be pinned down to one particular cause unless the person's entire life-style is looked at.

In some cases a patient 'not feeling too well' visits the doctor and asks for a tonic, when it is his way of living he should be considering.

Medical science has certainly not discovered all there is to know about curing the diseases that attack human beings. But it probably knows something about all of them.

If certain rules of health are followed, then many of the everyday ailments that upset our systems would in some cases be wiped out altogether and others reduced to a minimum. Which is why it is so important in the early training days of bringing up children that parents show wisdom. For the health of future generations rests on their good sense and good example.

EATING HABITS

Food is needed by the body for three reasons: *a) to supply heat to the body, b) to supply energy to the body, c) to repair body waste.*

Body heat is controlled by many factors, among them are local temperature, clothing, movement, the condition of the skin and tissue, especially the muscles and glands, chiefly the liver.

Even so, there is a daily loss to the body of about 2,500 calories of heat. This is lost by the skin, 77-80 per cent; by breathing, 17-20 per cent; by excreta, 3 per cent.

Air and food must supply the body with the chemicals needed by the tissues. These are: carbon, hydrogen, oxygen, calcium, nitrogen, sulphur, sodium potassium, magnesium, iron, phosphorus, chlorine and iodine. Food is made up of: proteins, fats, carbohydrates, vegetable acids, salts, vitamins and water. All are essential to health and growth. All are essential to life.

Carbohydrates. These include the monosaccharides, glucose, laevulose and galactose, which are found in the sweet juices of fruits, yeast, honey, etc.; the disaccharides, maltose, lactose and cane sugar, found in malt, milk, cane sugar and some plants, and the polysaccharides, including dextrine, starch glycogen and cellulose, which are found in beer, juices of most plants, crusts of bread, in seeds of cereals and potatoes, in liver, mussels and other tissues of animals.

Fats. A combination of trivalent alcohol (glycerin) with stearic, palmitic or oleic acid. Usually found in neutral fat in meat, oils, butter, cheese, cream, eggs, and nuts.

Mineral salts. Certain mineral salts need to be provided in definite amounts. Most common deficiency is in calcium, although iodine is often low in some people. You can get calcium in cheese, egg-yolk, milk, bran and green vegetables. Most of these also contain phosphorus, so does oatmeal. Iodine is found in fish, watercress, onion. Iron is found in egg-yolk, liver, oatmeal and green vegetables.

Proteins. These are vital for health and growth. The chief ones are: trytophane, tyrosine, cystine, lysine and arginine. Everyone needs a minimum of 37 grams a day.

Main sources of protein are from animal products, such as meat, cheese, eggs, milk and fish.

Vegetable acids. These contain sufficient oxygen to oxidise their hydrogen. They form carbonates for blood and other tissues, and are found in most vegetables.

Vitamins. These are classified in alphabetical order, and not according to what they do, as A, B complex (comprising B1, B2, B6 and other compounds), C, D, E and K.

Vitamin A is the anti-infective vitamin. If the body is deprived of it, septic complications can result. In adults, lack of it may produce softening of the cornea of the eyes. It is essential for forming tooth enamel, and for cell growth. It is present in fat, milk, butter, egg-yolk, cream, dried eggs, cod-liver oil, halibut oil, cheese, cabbage, potatoes, carrots, liver, kidney, heart, herring and salmon. The main source is from fish oils.

Vitamin B complex: Vitamin B1 is in cereals, eggs, yeast, malt, liver, kidney, potatoes and wholemeal. Pork muscle contains about eight times as much as beef. It is essential for the proper work of the starches. Lack of this vitamin effects the emotions and the nervous system. There is a loss of appetite, the individual becomes excessively tired however slight the exertion or mental effort, and suffers from vague, undefined gastro-intestinal disturbances.

If there is a big loss in this vitamin, the diseases that may result are Beri-beri and Polyneuritis, with enlargement of the heart. The body needs more during growth than in maturity.

Vitamin B2. An important source of B2 is egg-yolk, and in a lesser degree, in wholemeal bread, nuts, beans and peas. Partial deficiency can affect one's growth. The lips and mouth are also affected and the eyes may become inflamed. A marked deficiency produces a disease called

Pellagra, with a peculiar type of Eczema.

Vitamin B6 occurs in high concentration in seeds, yeast and liver. Shortage of this vitamin is responsible for insomnia, weakened muscles and cramp-like pains in the stomach.

Vitamin C is called ascorbic acid. There is plenty of it in fruits and fresh green vegetables. You need this vitamin to fight epidemics, particularly colds, 'flu, catarrh, and chest and respiratory diseases. At such times — but always, preferably — eat lots of oranges, grapefruit and lemons. They also prevent scurvy, and are essential for perfect health and development.

A deficiency of Vitamin C causes changes in the bones as well as dental diseases such as gingivitis, bleeding and swollen gums.

This vitamin is often lost in cooking. It is certainly destroyed by boiling green vegetables in soda, or carried away with the water they are cooked in. Vitamin C is present in fresh vegetables, such as cabbage, onions, swede, tomatoes; limes, oranges, lemons; raw meat juice; wheat, peas, lentils, beans (rolling or crushing will destroy the vitamins in these seeds). Orange juice is the richest source of Vitamin C.

Vitamin D is found in eggs, milk and in liver. The livers of many fish contain Vitamin D in large quantities. Loss of this vitamin leaves a person vulnerable to infections, especially of the chest and lungs. It plays a large part in the building up of lime and phosphorus in growing bones, and so is needed to counteract Rickets. This vitamin is effective in the growth and health of teeth and is vital to fight tooth decay.

Vitamin D is needed particularly by babies and young children. It can be built up in the body by the influence of sunshine or ultra-violet rays.

Fruit and vegetables get their Vitamin D content through exposure to the sun. It is also present in fat fish, especially fish liver oils, fish roe, egg-yolk, liver, whole wheat.

Vitamin E is necessary for fertility and reproduction. It prevents early sterility in both men and women. This vitamin is used to stimulate cattle breeding. It is found in oats, lettuce, meat, egg-yolk, liver, whole wheat.

Vitamin K. Leaves of plants contain this vitamin, which is so essential to man. A deficiency is characterised mainly

4

by haemorrhages, particularly in babies. It is responsible for certain allergic skin diseases, such as Urticaria, and some types of Alopecia (falling hair).

Normal Adult Diet
Personal preference plays a large part in the food we eat. But a diet should be a careful balance, to include: meat, fish, dairy products, eggs, fresh fruit, vegetables and water. You should get an adequate daily amount of:-

Protein (fish, meat, cheese, milk).

Fat, contained in oils cream and butter, etc.

Carbohydrates, contained in all forms of cereal, flour, cakes, bread, sugar, honey, syrup, etc.

Chemicals are covered sufficiently by a mixed diet.

Water. Drink plenty of it.

Vitamins.

Old people tend to concentrate, wrongly, on food that is easy to prepare and as a result often live on little more than bread, cakes and tea. They need iron in tablet form and vitamin capsules to reinforce their diet.

Special Diets
Bland diets: For those suffering with indigestion, an ulcer, or recovering from an illness, a special easily digested diet is necessary. *Food and drinks allowed are:-*

Milk and Eggs. Milk prepared in any way — junket, custard, well-cooked milk puddings, milk soup. Plain cream, made-up cream, ice-cream or cream soups. Butter. Eggs lightly cooked, beaten as egg and milk, or as custard.

Fish and Meat. Fish boiled, steamed, or baked, but not fried. Chicken or game roasted or baked. Tripe, brains, or sweetbread, well cooked, but not fried. Meat — beef or mutton occasionally, roasted or baked but not boiled or stewed.

Vegetables. Potatoes well cooked and mashed. Cauliflower, spinach, carrots, well cooked and rubbed through a sieve. Tomatoes fresh or cooked if rubbed through a sieve.

Fruit. If raw, avoid skins and pips. If cooked, always rub through a sieve: apricot fool, apple meringue, red currant, apple or marmalade jelly, damson cheese.

Various. White bread, cut thin and toasted dry. Any kind of smooth, plain biscuits. Plain sponge cakes, or light madeira cake without fruit. Jellies, plain chocolate,

5

honey and golden syrup.

Drinking. Drink sparingly with meals. You may take plenty of water between meals. Freshly-made weak tea, specially China tea, coffee with milk. Fruit juice. Milk. A small quantity of light wine is allowed with dinner or supper.

Meal instructions: Take your food regularly and avoid hurrying over it. Large meals are always bad. Frequent small meals should be your aim. Avoid taking a meal when you're tired or when you have cold hands or feet. Lie down, rest, and get warm first. Eat and chew thoroughly.

Food and drinks forbidden:

Fried foods.

Soups and meat dishes. *Avoid* meat soups and rich gravies; twice-cooked meat, sausages, made-up dishes, pork, 'high' game and all tough meat.

Fish. *Avoid* salmon, sardines, dried fish.

Condiments. *Avoid* spices, pepper, cayenne pepper, curries, vinegar, relishes, pickles, chutney and mustard.

Vegetables. *Avoid* cabbage, peas, beans, celery, onions, watercress, and cucumber; other vegetables must be passed through a sieve. You may add fresh butter to vegetables but don't cook them in fat. Avoid fried or chipped potatoes.

Fruit. *Avoid* all pips or skins of fruit (whether raw, cooked or in jam). Avoid raw apples, melon, marmalade, jam, lemon peel, currants, raisins, figs, nuts, and all unripe fruit.

Various. *Avoid* rich pastry or puddings, new bread, brown bread, porridge, and fruit cake. All cheese, other than cream cheese, is forbidden, and so is any cooked cheese.

Drinking. *Avoid* cocktails, spirits. Never take alcohol on an empty stomach. Avoid strong tea, black coffee and cocoa.

Smoking. Give up smoking if you have indigestion.

Anaemia diet: People with anaemia who are being treated by their doctor, taking iron tablets or having Vitamin B12 injections for Pernicious Anaemia, should follow this diet:-

Bread. Whole wheat.

Cereals. Preferably oatmeal, bran, shredded wheat.

Dairy products. As desired. At least one pint of milk a day.

Fruits. Preferably oranges, lemons, grapefruit, prunes, apricots.

Vegetables. All kinds, cooked and raw, especially spinach, peas, beans, cabbage, asparagus and lettuce.

Dessert. Fruits, milk puddings and plain desserts.

Meat. 1, Liver. 2, Red meats, roast beef, beef heart, steak. 3, Sweetbreads, kidney, brains. The last two can be substituted for liver.

Drinking. Tea, coffee, cocoa, Sanatogen, milk, fruit juices.

Take daily. 1, Two large servings of vegetables and fruits every meal. 2, Half a pound of liver or liver extract (directions are on the bottle).

Sample Menu.

Breakfast. Fruit, cereal. Egg and bacon. Brown bread and butter. Black treacle. Milk, ½ pint. Cream and sugar.

Lunch. Broth or vegetable soup. Meat. Potato. Vegetables (green or root). Bread and butter. Dessert.

Dinner. Cheese macaroni. Lettuce and tomato salad. Brown bread and butter. Fresh fruit. Sanatogen (2 teaspoons in ½ pint milk).

Low Residue diet: This is a diet for people suffering from intestinal disorders, colitis, Crohn's disease, etc. Foods allowed are:-

Bread. White (stale).

Cereals. Strained porridge and gruels.

Desserts. Custard, junkets, jellies, blancmange, milk puddings, plain cake.

Eggs. Lightly boiled, poached or scrambled.

Fruits. Sieved fruit, baked apple (without skin), ripe bananas. All pips, seed and skins must be removed.

Meats. Lamb, chicken and steamed fish.

Vegetables. Cooked and put through a sieve.

Soup. Strained vegetable soup.

Drinking. Cocoa, milk, Sanatogen, strained fruit juices, weak tea.

Sample Menu.

Breakfast. Strained porridge. Egg. Toast and butter. Sanatogen.

11.0 a.m. Orange juice and biscuits.

Lunch. Meat. Potato, mashed. Sieved vegetables. Egg

7

custard. Milk, one glass.

Tea. Bread and butter, honey or strained jam. Sponge cake or biscuit. Tea, milk, sugar.

Dinner. Strained vegetable soup. Steamed fish and sauce. Bread and butter. Apple sauce and junket.

At bedtime. Sanatogen, one cup.

Bland Purin-Free diet: This is for people suffering from high blood pressure, kidney trouble, gout, etc.

Sample Menu.

Breakfast. Fruit. Cereal. Egg. Toast and butter. Cup of Sanatogen.

Lunch. Boiled fowl or fish. Potato. Vegetables. Bread and butter. Dessert.

Tea. Bread and butter. Jam. Cake. Weak tea, milk, sugar.

Dinner. Cheese macaroni. Lettuce and tomato salad. Fruit. Plain cake or pudding. Cup of Sanatogen.

Foods to *avoid:* 1, Red and glandular meats. 2, Coffee, tea, cocoa, chocolate in excess. 3, Broths and meat soups. 4, Rich, highly seasoned food.

High Calorie diet: Anyone convalescing after an illness — or just wanting to put *on* weight — should follow this diet:-

Sample Menu.

Breakfast. Fruit. Cereal and cream. Bacon. Bread and butter. Marmalade or honey. Tea or coffee. One glass of milk.

11.0 a.m. 1 cup of Sanatogen (comprising 2 teaspoons Sanatogen, 1 tablespoon glucose, ¼ pint condensed milk).

Lunch. Milk soup, biscuits or toast. Meat. Potatoes (mashed with butter). Cooked vegetables. Dessert with cream. Bread and butter.

Tea. Bread and butter, jam. Cake. Tea, milk, sugar.

Dinner. Cheese omlette. Hot vegetable. Bread. Salad with mayonnaise. Fruit, junket, custard or cream. Cake. One glass of milk.

10.0 p.m. Cup of Sanatogen, made up as at 11.0 a.m.

To *increase* calories *add* the following to your food:-
1, Plenty of butter and cream. 2, Mayonnaise with salads. 3, Sugar and cream with food that needs it. 4, Sanatogen, made with condensed milk.

Reducing diet: For those who are overweight. *Don't* eat: sugar, cakes, pastries, puddings, jam, bread, potatoes, or fried food. *Do* eat plenty of fresh vegetables, salads, and all fresh fruit, *except* bananas.

Sample Menu.

Breakfast. Tea, milk (two tablespoons). Two eggs. 1 wheat biscuit or Ryvita. Butter (a piece the size of half a walnut). Tomatoes, ¼lb.

Lunch. Lean meat, or a good portion of cheese (about 3 ozs.). Lots of green vegetables or salad. 1 small apple, orange, pear or grapefruit.

Tea. Tea, milk (two tablespoons). 1 egg. 1 wheat biscuit or Ryvita. Butter (a piece the size of half a walnut).

Total. 1,128 calories.

Acid Stomach diet: Poor nutrition in children is often the result of digestive disturbances caused by too much acid in the system. The following are suggested:-

Protein foods (low in fat content): 1, Lean beef, lamb, liver, chicken. 2, Skimmed milk. 3, Steamed or boiled fish. 4, Eggs.

Puddings (low in fat content): 1, Jelly. 2, Fruit whip (made with egg white). 3, Blancmange (made with skimmed milk). 4, Skimmed milk pudding. 5, Cornflour and fruit juice combinations. 6, Fresh, dried and tinned fruit. 7, Sponge cake. 8, Fruit charlotte. 9, Custard. 10, Barley sugar.

Foods to *avoid:* 1, Fried foods. 2, Chocolates and toffee. 3, Pastry. 4, Nuts. 5, Cream and butter.

Sample Menu.

Breakfast. Fruit. Cereal and skimmed milk. Dry toast. Marmalade or honey. Sanatogen (½ pint skimmed milk).

Lunch. Lean meat. Potato. Vegetables. Blancmange and fruit.

Tea. Baked tomato on toast. Stewed fruit and sponge cake. Glass of skimmed milk.

Bedtime. Sanatogen, ¼ pint skimmed milk. Cold water, biscuit.

Before embarking on any of the diets described it is advisable to consult your family doctor.

THE EAR

Bleeding. This can happen after an accident or blow on the head. Get medical help immediately as it may be the sign of a fracture to the base of the skull.

Boil *(Furunculosis)*. This can happen through infection of a hair follicle or gland. It is caused by scratching the ear, or as a result of boils elsewhere in the body, or by chronic discharge of the middle ear.

In recurring boils of the ear, the urine should be tested by the doctor to eliminate any possible diabetic cause. If the boil doesn't rupture spontaneously, the doctor will prescribe an antibiotic.

Discharge from the Middle Ear *(Chronic Suppuration)*. A persistent nasal catarrh which has remained untreated, or adenoids, are the usual cause. Unhealthy surrounds and poor health can aggravate these conditions.

This condition may go on for years without any worry. Treatment, unfortunately, is not usually sought until deafness, headache, giddiness, neuralgia, or an increase in the discharge, causes the victim or parents' concern.

Treatment is not advised unless prescribed by a doctor, who should be consulted early in every case.

Ear Growth *(Polypus)*. This usually appears in the mucous membrane. There may be one or more, and they are usually a symptom of another disease. Treatment is by minor surgery by an ear specialist.

Eczema. If this occurs inside the ear, always consult a doctor. The condition may easily become chronic if not dealt with right away.

Foreign Bodies. Children often put beads and bits in their ears and forget about them. Adults sometimes forget cotton wool plugs. A foreign body, like a fly, pressing on the eardrum may cause deafness, noises in the head (Tinnitus), a dry cough and sometimes vomiting.

Don't meddle. Consult the doctor or an ear specialist.

Middle Ear. This includes the ear drum, the tympanic chamber, the three small bones called auditory ossicles —

the hammer, anvil and stirrup — and the Eustachian tube, which leads from mid ear to the back of the throat.

Acute inflammation of the middle ear may be caused by a severe cold in the head, nasal catarrh, the infectious fevers such as scarlet fever, measles, diphtheria or smallpox, or result from flu, pneumonia or whooping cough, from internal septic infections, or from head injuries.

Symptoms may vary according to the cause of the inflammation. Pain may be an occasional twinge or acute, continuous pain radiating from the ear up the side of the head. There may be temporary or intermittent deafness, noises in the head, a high temperature, possibly a discharge from the ear.

In children there may be convulsions and vomiting, for they suffer greater pain and may have a higher temperature than adults suffering from the same disorder. All earache in children is due to an inflamed eardrum and needs treating with antibiotics within 24 hours, if the hearing is not to be damaged.

Where there are repeated attacks of earache an ear, nose and throat specialist should be consulted, in case the tonsils and adenoids need to be removed.

Wax *(Cerumen).* This is secreted from glands in the outer ear. If excessive it can vary from a semi-solid mass to a hard plug of grey or black wax.

This occurs because either the glands are over secreting or soap is continually being left behind after washing. If the wax is hard, soften either with warm olive oil or glycerine drops inserted in the ear two or three times a day for a few days. Then it can be syringed, but not by an amateur. Far better to get a doctor to do it. Remember, the ears are delicate.

Glossary
AUDITORY: Sense of hearing.
AUDITORY CANAL: *Outer:* Passage from the outer meatus to the tympanic membrane or ear drum. *Inner:* Passage in the petrous bone for the hearing and facial nerves and the auditory blood vessels.
AURICLE: The ear outside the head.
CERUMEN: Ear wax.
DEAFNESS: *Labyrinthine:* Associated with the middle ear.

Family degenerative: A hereditary condition of labyrinthine deafness. *Old age:* Usually accompanies hardening of the arteries. A labyrinthine type. *Syphilitic:* Occurs in acquired and hereditary syphilis. *Toxic:* A labyrinthine type caused by poisons acting on the auditory nerve. *Congenital:* Due to bad development of the middle ear. *Boilermaker's:* Caused by working in places where sound is deafening. *Hysterical:* Appears and disappears with the hysteria in affected patients. *Music:* Inability to identify musical notes (tone deafness); *Vascular:* Due to a disease of the blood vessels of the ear.

EUSTACHIAN TUBE: A tube one-and-a-half to two inches long extending from the naso-pharynx to the eardrum. Its purpose is to equalise the pressure between the eardrums and the outer air. If blocked causes deafness with noises in the outer ear *(Tinnitus Aurium).*

HEARING: Sound waves travel through the outer ear to the drum, which vibrates. These vibrations are transmitted across the middle ear by the three little bones, the hammer, the anvil and the stirrup, to the internal ear. Then to the ends of the auditory nerves and to the brain.

INNER EAR — or LABYRINTHINE: This is embedded in the petrous portion of the temporal bone, and contains three semi-circular canals and other delicate structures, the nerve endings of the eighth cranial nerves — the auditory nerve (or nerve of hearing).

MASTOID PROCESS: The nipple-shaped portion of the temporal bone lying immediately behind the ear, containing large air spaces communicating with the middle ear.

MASTOID: From the Greek 'nipple-shaped'.

MENIERE'S DISEASE: A disease of the inner ear causing giddiness and deafness, with noises in the ear. The giddiness is known as vertigo and the patient's sense of balance may be temporarily affected.

MIDDLE EAR: The cavity on the inner side of the eardrum and communicating with the outer air via the Eustachian tube.

OTTIS MEDIA: Inflammation of the middle ear.

TYMPANIC MEMBRANE: Eardrum.

THE EYES
Care of the Eyes. Never abuse the eyes. Our sight is the most important, valuable and intricate of all the senses.

Parents should be jealous of the sight of their children and never hesitate to seek advice if it is needed. The use of glasses to correct a fault in a young child may avoid a need for glasses at a later stage in life.

Always, at any age, seek specialist advice before obtaining glasses. Special treatment of an eye condition may possibly correct a fault without permanent need for spectacles.

The science of orthoptics is the method of correction of eye defects by special exercises.

For those whose eyes may be exposed to undue strain, working long hours in artificial light, or on close and detailed indoor work, special care is essential. Cold eye pads applied to tired eyes give great relief.

Because the human eye is so sensitive, it is important that eye lotions should be non-irritant, mildly antiseptic and physically compatible with the normal tear solution bathing the eye.

Treatment for tired, strained eyes: A simple saline made with distilled water is helpful. A 10 per cent distilled extract of witch hazel added to the above lotions will soothe and have a cooling, astringent effect.

Black Eye *(Ecchymosis of the Eyelids)*. Cotton wool or lint soaked in cold water bandage, or even ice in an appropriately padded cloth, will check the swelling and discolouration.

The skin should never be punctured no matter how large the swelling. If the condition is severe, or if the eyeball is itself damaged, the doctor should be consulted.

Cataract. This condition usually occurs in men and women in their late fifties, early sixties. The eye vision is blocked by milky opacity which occurs in the lens of the eye. An eye surgeon can remove the opaque lens, when it is 'ripe', and fit the patient with spectacles to compensate for the lack of sight.

Conjunctivitis. Inflammation of the delicate membrane which lines the eyelids and covers the eyeball. Sometimes this condition can be accompanied by a discharge. It should never be ignored, particularly in new born babies. Before treatment is given, correct diagnosis should be made either by a doctor or at an eye hospital.

Inversion of the Lower Lid. This sometimes happens in old people. A doctor should always be called, as it may lead to ulceration of the cornea.

Squint. Curable in most cases today by the progress of ophthalmology. Mothers should never delay getting early advice and treatment for their children. A child may develop a squint after whooping cough. A watchful mother will notice and should seek advice at the slightest sign.

Stye. Inflammation of one of the sebaceous glands of the eyelids, or infection of the hair follicle of the eyelash.

If it is small and not painful, apply hot pads to the area concerned. The stye may be dispersed quite quickly. If the affected eyelash is pulled out the pus will discharge and the condition clear. A large or painful stye should be treated by a doctor or eye specialist. A Chloromycetin eye ointment is helpful.

Watering, painful eyes. This condition may be due to in-growing eyelashes, which should only be removed by a doctor. But it usually indicates a foreign body in the eye, such as grit or dust, which should be removed if obvious with a small piece of clean lint, the corner of a clean hanky, or a fine camel-hair brush.

If the foreign body cannot be removed easily, consult a doctor or eye hospital, to prevent possible injury to the eyeball.

Glossary

ASTIGMATISM. A defect of the curvature of the refractive surfaces of the eye, so that the rays of light are not focused on a single point.

BLEPHARITIS. Inflammation of the eyelid.

CATARACT. Transparency of the lens is lost to a greater or lesser degree.

EMMETROPIA. From the Greek, 'in proper measure vision'. The normal condition of the eye with perfect vision, it is the perfect type of eye. Any variation from this is called:

AMETROPIA. From the Greek, 'irregular eye'.

GLAUCOMA. The result of raised tension of the fluid within the eyeball.

HORDEOLUM. A stye.

HYPERMETROPIA. Far-sightedness. The hypertropic eye is the undeveloped eye in which parallel rays of light come to focus behind the retina. Consequently, this type of eye, if at rest, sees everything indistinctly. Eye-strain is a common and predominant symptom. Corrected by convex lenses.

MYOPIA. Short-sightedness.

NYCTALOPIA. Night blindness.

OPHTHALMIA. Severe inflammation of the eye or of the conjunctiva.

OPHTHALMOLOGIST. A trained eye specialist skilled in the diseases of the eye.

OPTICIAN. A maker or seller of glasses.

PRESBYOPIA. From the Greek 'old eye'. Long sight and impairment of vision due to old age. The power of accommodation is diminished due to loss of the elasticity of the lens, so that the near point of distinct vision is removed farther from the eye.

REFRACTION. Testing the eyes for errors of vision.

RETINA. The sense organ of vision at the back of the eye, connected to the optic nerve.

STRABISMUS. Squint.

HEADACHE

Headache is not a disease in itself. It is a symptom of another disorder. While aspirin may cure the pain, the patient should always remember that the cause of the headache, whether it is infrequent or persistent, must be diagnosed correctly, and treated accordingly. These are some of the more usual causes of headache:

Eyestrain. Pain in this case may be felt at the front of the head and behind the eyes. The sufferer may show it by wrinkling the brow to focus the eyes properly. Frowning often accompanies such a headache, and is often associated with a tired and burning feeling of the eyeballs.

Don't hesitate to consult a fully qualified ophthalmic specialist for treatment, and possibly glasses.

Disease or Disorder of the Ear, Nose and Throat. Breathing through the mouth in cases of adenoids or enlarged tonsils; a blocked nose passage; a cold; sinus trouble; blocking of the external ear passage because of too much wax or a foreign body in the ear. All or any of these may cause a headache. The site of the pain is usually over the forehead.

If the headache persists, see a doctor so that the cause of the headache can be diagnosed and treated.

Fatigue. Someone who has overworked physically may be so worn out that his head aches. But so will someone who has overdone it by sitting behind his desk worrying over some figures. Rest is the only cure.

Nervous Headaches. These occur in cases of migraine, epilepsy and other nervous complaints. They should be regarded as chronic and part of the disease but they must still be checked on and the cause treated.

Organic head and body disorders. A blow on the head, fever, a tumour will produce headaches; sometimes severe ones. So will blood disorders such as anaemia and high blood-pressure. See a doctor at once if you have a bad, persistent or recurring headache.

Poisons. A heavy feeling in the head, or severe headache, can be caused by what is in the atmosphere, such as a badly ventilated room, someone's over-indulgence in tobacco, alcohol, drugs, fumes from petrol, coal gas, paint, coke, or other similar substances.

Remove the cause, get into the fresh air, and your headache should soon disappear.

Constipation and disorders of the kidneys may produce headache. Also headache may accompany a woman's monthly period.

Teeth. Bad teeth, including wisdom teeth (at the back of the jaw) often cause headache in grown-ups. The pain is usually at the back of the head. See the dentist for treatment, and possibly an X-ray.

Never disregard a headache, in a child or adult. It is not normal, but a sign of ill health in one form or another.

Treatment: If the headache is rare, slight and cannot be attributed to any particular origin, take one of the following:

Aspirin, Veganin (good for monthly periods), Panadol. Two tablets every four hours for adults, but don't keep on taking them for weeks on end. *With a persistent headache, see a doctor.*

HEALTH AND TRAVEL

Most leading airlines have medical departments where people with certain medical conditions can check that they are fit enough to fly. Special oxygen equipment can be provided, though it *is* safer to check first, both from your health point of view and the availability of the equipment.

But it is far more sensible for anyone planning a long journey — whether by air, ship, train or car — to consult their own doctor beforehand.

Some people are simply bad travellers and get headaches and tummy upsets at the slightest tilt of a plane, lurch of a ship or jolt in a car.

However, there are many men and women who love travelling, but whose poor health can be accelerated by flying, sailing, motoring or going on a train journey.

People with the following conditions should certainly consult their own doctor and/or the air or shipping line *before* booking a ticket:

Blood Diseases. Any blood condition which reduces the number of red blood cells to under 2½ million per cubic millimetre, or the haemoglobin to under 50 per cent, or cause a tendency to haemorrhages, cannot fly without oxygen. The patient may need a blood transfusion before the journey.

It is advisable in such a case to consult the airline's medical officer before the trip is booked.

Chest Diseases. Air travel is particularly hard on anyone with an acute head cold or temporary blockage of the ear drums.

Asthma, bronchitis, emphysema (enlargement of the air sacs of the lungs, a chronic condition affecting the breathing), and fibroid lung are not helped, and can be accelerated, by air travel. Particularly if the patient is permanently short of breath. *If* they are allowed to fly, oxygen must be made available.

Any case of active tuberculosis cannot be carried while the condition is still rated infectious.

Other lung conditions may need oxygen. But each case must be judged on how severe it is, and how breathless the patient is likely to get.

Gastro-intestinal Disease. The reduced pressure of air travel, aggravated by air sickness, can cause a gastric or duodenal ulcer to bleed or perforate. Anyone with this condition should definitely not fly until a month after recovering from a bleed, whether it is coughed up from the stomach or passed out in the motions.

It is very unwise to fly until at least two weeks after any abdominal operation. Sensibly, leave travel for a month in such circumstances. And check with your doctor.

The person who wants to travel but is doubtful about his condition, should also check with the airline medical officer about his suitability to travel. *No chances should be taken.*

Heart Diseases. Those suffering with angina or a heart condition which is being treated, and regulated, by a doctor, and who cannot exercise without becoming out of breath, should mention this to the airline's medical officer. Special oxygen breathing equipment will be made available, if possible, just in case of an emergency.

Patients with heart failure and who may develop severe breathing difficulties will have to be considered by the airline medical officer. He *may* decide the patient is not well enough to travel, but he may make oxygen equipment available.

Anyone who has had a coronary thrombosis should not fly until he has been free of all symptoms for two to three months. Patients with high blood pressure should have a sedative before the flight. Extra oxygen should be made available. But in all such cases consult your own doctor, and inform the airline *before* you take off.

Inoculation. Today many countries have tightened up and laid down compulsory health laws — such as vaccination against smallpox. If the traveller is going to, or through the yellow fever areas of the world, then those countries 'on the way' insist on immunisation against yellow fever too.

The traveller has to realise the difference between which inoculations are compulsory and which are desirable. A passenger will not be allowed to land from his plane and may waste a lot of time having to be inoculated and injected — unless he has received the compulsory inoculations beforehand.

International Sanitary Regulations specify the following periods for the validity of International Certificates for compulsory inoculations:

Type of Vaccination	Certificate valid for	Period validity begins
Smallpox		
Primary vaccination	3 years	8 days later
Re-vaccination	3 years	At once
Cholera		
Primary vaccination	6 months	6 days later
Re-vaccination within six months	6 months	At once
Yellow Fever		
Primary vaccination	6 years	10 days later
Re-vaccination after six years	6 years	At once

These rules vary from country to country and from year to year so it would be sensible to make enquiries early regarding the current rules in force, not only in the country of your destination but those through which you're going to travel.

These International Certificates, in blank form, have to be obtained by the traveller and taken to the doctor for completion. Afterwards they must be taken to the local medical officer of health to be stamped, before they will be accepted abroad.

The blank forms can be obtained from the travel agency or airline or direct from one of the following:

Department of Health and Social Security, Elephant and Castle, London, SE1.

Welsh Board of Health, Cathays Park, Cardiff.

Scottish Home and Health Department, St. Andrew's House, Edinburgh, 1.

Nervous Disorders. Lack of oxygen and a struggle for air can aggravate the condition of people suffering with uncontrolled epilepsy. Those with impaired mentality might be allowed to travel, if they are sedated or accompanied by someone.

Pregnancy. Most airlines will let expectant mothers (up to the 32nd. week) travel. On short internal air trips the rule may be relaxed a little. This restriction is enforced to avoid the risk of a confinement when airborne.

Women who are liable to miscarry should not fly until after the third month, in case a bumpy journey precipitates the start of a miscarriage.

MENOPAUSE

Today, the change of life — so often dreaded by women and dismissed by doctors in 'grin and bear it' terms — is being treated in a more enlightened fashion both physically and psychologically.

Progressive-minded doctors, and even the local GP round the corner, are beginning to realise the importance of hormone treatment to ease a woman through the menopause, while also possibly prolonging her youth and good health.

Menopause clinics are being set up in hospitals, and as separate units, throughout the country.

The menopause — the period when menstruation slows down and stops — usually occurs between the ages of 45 and 50. It may start as early as 40 and as late as 52. Some healthy women continue having periods until they are 55 years old. The change can last from six months to three years. The age it starts often follows that of a woman's mother.

A train of events is set in motion at the onset, when egg cells are no longer released from the ovaries. At the same time the ovaries drastically reduce their production of the femal sex hormone, oestrogen.

As menstruation stops, so the body must adapt to a new hormone balance, which explains why a woman gets minor physical and psychological disturbances, such as sudden high temperatures known as hot flushes (especially of the face and neck), lasting from one to several minutes and followed by cold sweats. These may be accompanied by nausea, uncontrollable irritability, dizziness, especially on stopping or looking up suddenly, and depression.

These symptoms vary from one woman to another, in number and severity. Many women become fatter, and early arthritis of the knees is noticeable, particularly in the working woman who is a cleaner or waitress, or simply a dedicated housewife.

It is dangerous for any woman to accept that the change of life usually starts with a lot of menstrual bleeding or flooding. If this happens at any time during the menopause or afterwards, she should at once seek medical or gynaecological advice.

Many women sail through the menopause without great stress. Others don't. Some women experience emotional turmoil and a feeling they are no longer feminine. Others find their sexual feelings do not stop during or after the change. Certainly, many women benefit from some form of oestrogen treatment, or the more sophisticated hormone replacement therapy (H.R.T.). But a woman must put pressure on her old-fashioned doctor who often traditionally feels she should just put up with 'the change'.

There are menopause clinics at the following: *Aberdeen University; Queen Elizabeth Medical Centre, Birmingham; the Royal Sussex Hospital, Brighton; Southmead Hospital, Bristol; Royal Infirmary, Edinburgh; Dryburn Hospital, Durham; Glasgow Royal Infirmary; General Infirmary, Leeds; King's College Hospital, Dulwich Hospital, Chelsea Hospital for Women, St. Thomas's Hospital, all in London; City Hospital, Nottingham; George Eliot Hospital, Nuneaton; John Radcliffe Hospital, Oxford; Jessop Hospital, Sheffield; St. Tydfil's Hospital, Merthyr Tydfil.*

MENSTRUATION

This is the monthly bleeding from the womb *(uterus)* in women of child-bearing age — that is from the age of 9 to 14 to about 50.

Menstruation is one stage of a constantly repeated cycle, in which the lining of the womb (the *endometrium)* repeatedly becomes swollen with extra blood and tissue. This is the body's preparation to receive a fertilised egg cell *(ovum)* from the ovaries. The process is controlled by the pituitary gland and the ovaries.

On the first day of menstruation, at the start of the cycle, an egg cell grows in an ovary. It continues growing for 14 days. When ripe, and about the size of a pea, it bursts and the egg enters the Fallopian tube on its way to the womb. If it is fertilised in the next five or six days by meeting a male sperm cell, it becomes implanted in the lining of the womb. Menstruation then stops for nine months, the duration of the pregnancy. Those five or six days, which vary according to the length of the cycle and a woman's age, are what is known as a woman's 'danger period'. The peak time for conception.

If the egg isn't fertilised, it is discharged from the vagina in the menstrual flow.

First Menstruation Period. The 'period' or 'curse', as women refer to it, lasts from three to six days. The amount of bleeding depends on her general health and work.

Over the past 20 years or so girls in our highly civilised society have started to mature earlier. They start their monthly periods now more often at 10 to 12 than the old average, 13 to 14. However, this can fluctuate widely, according to race and amongst members of the same race. It can start as low as 9 and as late as 18 or 19. When it develops late it is because of delayed growth of the womb.

If a girl gets severe pain and excessive bleeding, she should be seen by her doctor as these conditions can be helped by drugs, vitamins, or in rare cases, a small operation.

Menstruation varies in other ways. In one woman it can occur every 25 days, in others every 30 days — though the average is 28 days. During the period a woman uses either an external sanitary towel or internal Tampon to absorb the blood.

Just before the monthly period the fluid-salt balance in the body is disturbed. A woman can be depressed, emotionally tense and suffer headaches, signs to her that her period is imminent. Her skin may be a bit puffy in the abdomen and other parts of the body, her breasts tingle, and she may frequently put on a pound or two in weight — though this soon disappears as the period ends.

Disturbances in Menstruation. There are three main causes:
Amenorrhoea. The periods may be absent or very sparse or very occasional. This may be as a result of pregnancy, breast-feeding, shock, change of climate, or a symptom of anaemia, tuberculosis, or even a congenital condition preventing the proper exercise of the sex organs. In all cases a woman should see her doctor for treatment.

Dysmenorrhoea. Painful periods are experienced by many women. But pain handicaps only a few. Such cases shouldn't be considered normal, and the woman should go to her doctor. Drugs, a change of diet or routine, or even a slight operation, may put the matter right. Modern gynaecology has made great strides in the past few years in treating this condition. Women vary in their tolerance to pain and the psychological approach is as important as the physical. In many cases dysmenorrhoea disappears after childbirth, as the dilation of the uterine canal relieves the congestion or spasm which originally caused the pain.

Menorrhagia. This is excessive loss of blood during the period, and *metrorrhagia* is loss between the periods. Both are often caused by the same condition. Fibroids in the womb is the commonest cause. Sometimes it is because of upset of the hormones, the sequel to a miscarriage and any form of ulceration within the womb.

Heavy blood loss at *any time* justifies seeking medical help immediately.

SKIN, HAIR and NAILS
Abnormalities of the Hair. All hair is subject to seasonal fluctuations, a little natural 'shedding' in the spring or autumn. Or if a person is a bit run down, or recently recovered from an illness.

A common disorder causing falling hair, and often subsequent baldness, is seborrhoea of the scalp. It is first made obvious by white scales known as dandruff. The head is often itchy and scurfy.

Mild dandruff can be effectively treated by the better medicated shampoos available in hairdressers and shops. But if dandruff persists, and the hair is beginning to fall out profusely, don't hesitate to see your doctor and he will no doubt advise you to consult a trichologist, a specialist in these problems.

Abnormally oily skin *(Seborrhoea).* Sebum is the secretion of the skin's sebaceous (oil producing) glands and is chiefly composed of fat. Seborrhoea is not a disease, but it is unpleasant cosmetically' because of the oily shine it gives the face or the scalp, causing greasy hair. Young people are the most common sufferers and they quite often get dandruff too. Usually the condition disappears when they are out of their teens.

Treatment lies in removing whatever it is that accelerates the condition, such as cold, heat, light, wind, and weather. Try to remove the sebum from the skin by washing frequently, or by using a proprietary solvent containing spirit. A dusting powder of sulphur (5 per cent) and talcum, is very helpful.

When there is dandruff too a cream containing 4 per cent precipitated sulphur and 12 per cent of precipitated coal tar is very useful.

Acne. Puberty, plus too much oil secreted from the sebaceous glands, and constipation, are thought to make people extra sensitive to this unsightly skin infection. Irregular monthly periods, infected tonsils and teeth, may aggravate it. The earliest sign is a blackhead. But, in fact, the actual cause of acne is not really known.

In acne, a small raised spot may appear at the mouth of the skin gland. If the contents of the spot erupt to the surface, it may heal spontaneously. But it is quite usual for the spot to go down without breaking, and again fill up with pus. The acne may be cleared after coming to a head, by expressing it gently so as not to form a scar. Remember to heat the area first with hot water to open the pores.

Treatment: Wash with a super-fatted sulphur soap with resorcin. After washing, treat with a sulphur lotion. If there are lots of the spots, your doctor may prescribe antibiotic treatment. An acne vaccine is helpful, and internally, lots of Vitamin B1.

Birthmark *(Naevus).* This is a blemish on the skin at birth and it develops before the baby is born. The cause is unknown. If they are disfiguring, certain types can be removed by surgery, shrunk by injections, treated with dry ice or simply concealed by special cosmetics. But in any case this must always be done *medically,* and not by self-help treatment.

Most common are the dark red 'raspberry' and 'strawberry' birthmarks, and these are really an enlarged group of blood vessels in the skin. 'Portwine' type stains, another type of blood vessel birthmark, present a greater problem. Skin specialists, however, have developed various methods of making them look less conspicuous.

Blackheads *(Comedones).* If the skin glands become blocked in any way by secretion the result, almost always, is a blackhead. Cause is often, as with acne, a disturbance in the diet, constipation, puberty, and possibly not washing the

24

skin often enough with good old soap and water.

Similar *treatment* as that for acne. Blackheads can be squeezed out. But always remember to open the pores as much as possible by applying warm or hot water, or towels wrung out in hot water. The towels must be clean, preferably sterile.

With lots of difficult blackheads, it is best to see a doctor. If the complaint crops up again and again, with your doctor's advice, get a pair of comedo forceps from the chemist. They do help prevent unnecessary damage to the skin, if used with great care.

Care of the Hands. A normal skin keeps healthy and supple through the natural oil from the grease glands. Anything which de-greases the skin leaves it dry and brittle and liable to crack.

All detergents, furniture polish, oven cleaners, lavatory powders, pot scourers, turpentine, petrol, lime, cement, nail polish removers, etc. dry the skin. So protective gloves should be worn when handling these products.

For those who like to keep the skin and hands especially soft and supple, here is a hand lotion, often used after scrubbing up by surgeons:

> Tragacanth powder, 3 gns.
> Simple tincture of benzoin, 4 ml.
> Glycerine, 150 ml.
> Water to 600 ml.

Ask the chemist if he will colour it pink and add some eau-de-Cologne to make it smell nice. Rub a little into the hands each time after washing.

Cosmetics. There is nothing to beat soap and water, but protection is often necessary for the skin, as well as the enhancement of a woman's best features. This is why most modern skin make-up is milder and moisturiser-based.

Sun is a beauty giver, if used wisely and not too much. It produces Vitamin D when reacting on the skin secretions, so is very beneficial to the health. Where there is no sun, or it is too weak to have much effect, ultra-violet light or quartz light can be used as artificial aids. This method of irradiation is useful in such diseases as rickets, diabetes, tuberculosis of the skin, and in inducing sleep.

Too much sun is dangerous, which is why the enthusiastic

sun-bather must do it in short daily stints, starting with five minutes and gradually increasing. Use protective lotions or creams if the sun is very hot.

Dilated or Enlarged Pores *(Megaloporia)*. These are most often found on and around the nose. Careful *treatment* by an ultra-violet lamp — under strict supervision — can bring relief and improvement. But the only real cure is to have the surrounding skin removed by a plastic surgeon.

Eczema. This condition may occur if the skin is especially oily or dry. It can be very tormenting in young children, who become irritable and restless. Many children affected have a family history of allergies, such as bronchial trouble, asthma or hay fever. Repeated use of harsh detergents and domestic powders may cause it, or the sufferer may be allergic to such things as paint, rubber, or even barbiturate drugs.

In eczema the skin goes red and there are blisters and an itchy rash. Often the skin crusts and scales. Some types clear up spontaneously.

Treatment by sedatives and hydrocortisone skin cream can be rapidly effective in most cases. In the acute stages, a soothing oily calamine lotion is advisable. Ointments should *not* be used. If they are used without medical knowledge they may increase the inflammation, irritation and discharge.

If the sufferer has dyspepsia or constipation these must be treated. Alcohol and highly seasoned food should be avoided, especially when eczema accompanies gout. If it is present on the legs as varicose eczema, any varicose veins must receive treatment. Eczema is not infectious.

Heavy Sweating *(Hyperhydrosis)*. Excessive perspiration varies in intensity and also in type. Sometimes the entire skin is affected, sometimes just certain areas.

If sweat isn't allowed to evaporate, it decomposes and gives off an offensive smell and may ruin clothes. Body sweat is most prevalent under the armpits and in the feet. It can be cold, or hot, and may be caused by another bodily disorder or simply by over-active sweat glands in a certain part of the body. If it is persistent and profuse, as with any disorder, a doctor should be consulted and treatment will be given.

Frequent bathing is essential for personal freshness, and frequent changes of clothes are vital for someone who perspires heavily. The girl who tends to sweat beneath the arms should bathe daily and have a fresh dress or blouse on every day; the man with a tendency to sweaty feet should not only have fresh socks each day, but a change of shoes.

Treatment: Apart from those anti-perspirants and deodorants that can be bought in the shops — and among the dozens of varieties there must be one to suit everybody — there are remedies that can be made up by the chemist. The best is a 30 per cent solution of formalin in tap water, or a 10 per cent solution of aluminium chloride. The best powders contain salicylic acid or tannoform mixed with a talc base.

A useful prescription for a powder for tender feet, which are caused by heavy sweating, is: Potash alum, 15 parts; Talc in fine powder, 85 parts.

Impetigo. A highly contagious skin disease. It is most common in children and usually appears on the face. Sometimes men with beards get it, and it is popularly known as 'Barber's Rash'. It surfaces with a blister which breaks after the first hour or after a day or so. The blister may produce a thick yellow crusty type pus, or thin and almost colourless. The incubation period is three days.

As it is so infectious it may quickly spread to the scalp or other parts of the body, particularly through scratching or use of towels. Sometimes impetigo is mistaken for weeping eczema or ringworm, but the doctor will know the difference, and it should clear up in about three weeks, though some cases take much longer.

Treatment: Modern antibiotics, such as aureomycin, applied as ointment and swallowed as tablets, are highly effective.

Milium. Hard whiteish deposits, each about the size of a grain of sand, which lie close under the skin. Don't fiddle with them yourself as you may break the skin.

Treatment should be left to a doctor, who will split the skin properly and squeeze these deposits out.

Mole. Moles are dark spots of pigment in the skin — some are blue or even white, but mostly they are brown. Sometimes they are raised and hairs grow from them.

Never, never pick at a mole or try to cut one off. In rare cases, not noticeable until put under a microscope, they can be malignant.

If a mole bleeds, gets bigger or darker, see a doctor and a specialist. Irritable moles can be removed surgically, so can conspicuous ones. But specialist attention is vital in such cases.

Nails. Some diseases of the skin, such as Eczema, may have a bad effect on the nails. White spots may be ignored. Furrows running across the nails may be the result of poor circulation. This must be treated before the nails can be improved.

If the nails are soft, then this shows a lack of calcium in the diet. So eat lots more eggs, cheese, milk, bran and green vegetables. Watch for an improvement and consult your doctor if the problem persists, as you may have an imbalance in the system.

Whitlows, an inflammation at the base of the nail, can be most painful and look unsightly. These are best treated by your doctor.

Psoriasis. Skin eruptions in the form of itchy red patches, covered with loose, silvery scales, which appear most often on the arms, legs, knees, elbows, scalp; sometimes on the chest, stomach and back and soles of the feet. Psoriasis is sometimes linked with arthritis. It can be acute but is usually chronic and mild. There is no foolproof cure.

Treatment by steriod drugs applied to the affected area is fairly effective. A doctor will prescribe ointments and lotions to ease the itching and heal the skin lesions.

Many people find that sensible exposure to sunlight and the sun is slightly beneficial during the summer. But sunburn is certainly *not*.

Psoriasis sufferers in this country can get advice and information from The Psoriasis Association, 22 Billing Road, Northampton, NN1 5AT.

Skin Disorders and treatments for the Face and Neck. Skin problems are often worsened by ill-advised home treatment and the use of medicines without medical guidance. Always see a doctor about a skin complaint if you want to see a quick recovery.

Superfluous Hair *(Hypertrichosis).* This is when fine body hairs, usually barely noticeable, develop into hairs of ordinary size and thickness.

To destroy a hair like this it is necessary to get to the hair follicle which lies well below the surface and put that out of action.

Clearly, hair remover advertisements which declare they *can* remove hair permanently, *cannot.* The product or method will only remove the hair which appears above the surface. The only safe and permanent method is electrolysis, and this must be employed by an expert who has the special skill and knowledge. That expert must also be *qualified.*

Sometimes the growth of superfluous hair is so excessive it may be associated with disease of the suprarenal gland, in which case consult your doctor.

SLEEP

What is it and how much do we need? Sleep is very much a mystery despite the fact that we have been enjoying it since the beginning of time, and despite the vast amount of research done on it.

Sleep is essential to mental and physical fitness and health. It is a voluntary state of rest during which a person's body and nervous system become almost inactive. The conscious mind stops functioning and only our breathing and digestion continue.

A newborn baby sleeps most of the day, waking only for feeds; a young child needs 11 to 12 hours' sleep; most adults manage well with six to eight hours — eight hours being most usual. Some can stay fit and healthy on two hours, while others moan if they get less than 10 hours.

Many people who complain of *insomnia* (the inability to sleep) do not in fact need more sleep than they are getting.

Average hours of sleep needed by children:

Age	Hours needed
6 months	18
1 year	14 to 16
2 years	12 to 14
5 years	10 to 12
10 years	10 to 11
16 years	9

Teenagers, with so many pursuits such as parties, dancing, sport, all vying for their attention, rarely today get the nine hours sleep they need each night. Many of them fight off sleep by drinking strong black coffee or one of the soft drinks claimed by the manufacturers to give 'life'. These contain caffeine citrate, a brain stimulant, and the active ingredient of strong black coffee.

Some of these young people, in their efforts to keep going, succumb to taking pep pills, little realising that this is often the first step on the road to drug addiction and all its horrifying consequences.

Factors Encouraging Normal Sleep

Mental peace and contentment, physical tiredness, warmth, fresh air, pleasant surroundings and a comfortable bed are all conducive to sleep, while pain anxiety, noise and lack of warmth will effectively keep you awake.

Bedclothes and Warmth. Snuggling down into a warm, comfy bed is a luxury that can make you feel sleepy just thinking about it, but it is important to remember that heavy bedclothes are not necessarily warmer than light-weight coverings. Really heavy blankets do in fact cause some people to have violent dreams.

In the last few years the continental quilt, or duvet, has become so popular it is now a top chain store-seller. The duvet is a lightweight quilt, filled either with goose, goose and duck feathers, or Terylene. It can be bought with attractive covers, matching pillows, toning sheets and, for the housewife, it is a great time saver. For it really incorporates a top sheet, blanket and eiderdown, and certainly makes bed-making easier.

The duvet is probably not the warmest bed covering. But for young couples, particularly, it is cosy and warm in winter, and cool in summer.

For a *really* warm bed there is little to beat the electric blanket, so beloved by the older generation. Electric blankets are designed to give a pre-determined degree of heat. So unless they are used strictly to the manufacturer's instructions they can be dangerous.

The body normally sweats during sleep. Obviously the warmer a person is the more he will sweat. If someone sleeps on a switched-on blanket that is not thermostatically controlled — and manufacturers warn against this — there is the very real danger that sweat will seep into the blanket. This will alter the electrical resistance and cause it to become so overheated a heavy sleeper may well suffer burns.

There are even greater dangers for people with diseases likely to cause coma (diabetes and epilepsy for instance), bed-wetting or any other illness which may make even a thermostatically controlled blanket become moist. Recently there have been many cases of burns from this cause.

No electric blanket should be left on during sleep. Not only should it be switched off but the mains plug should be removed from its socket.

Fatigue and Supper Time Drinks. If your body isn't tired, then obviously it is not ready for sleep. Just to go to bed at a fixed time through habit will only result in insomnia. Those who are not tired as bedtime approaches, and who can't stay up until the small hours, may find a long walk after supper will tire them out. A warm bath before bed is very relaxing and entices sleep.

Older people often sleep badly in the night. This is sometimes because they have cat-naps during the day and may have taken very little exercise. As alcohol is a sedative, a hot toddy containing whisky or rum immediately before going to bed may help them sleep. If that doesn't work it may be necessary to get a mild sedative from the doctor.

Coffee contains caffeine citrate, a brain stimulant, and is not a good bed-time drink. Nor, contrary to what most people believe, is cocoa, because it induces the kidneys to work faster. Any type of drink taken late at night disturbs some people, particularly poor sleepers. So they should either do without a supper time drink, or put up with the inconvenience of visiting the toilet in the early hours and the difficulty of getting back to sleep.

Freedom from Pain, Anxiety and Depression. Pain and anxiety both prevent sleep. So once the causes have been removed the insomnia problem disappears.

Depression *and* insomnia are a different matter. It indicates that the sufferer is in need of medical advice, because this is often the start of a mental imbalance that could lead to a suicide attempt. Many people like this are so mentally sick they won't seek medical help, in which case it is the responsibility of relatives to consult a doctor for them.

The Mattress. A good mattress must support the body and keep the spine flat, as well as allowing the muscles to relax. If a mattress doesn't give this sort of support it encourages the spine to become curved. This means one set of spinal muscles is stretched, the others bunched up and cramped.

Because people come in all shapes and sizes it is obvious no one type of spring mattress will suit everybody. A mattress that suits a wife's eight stone will be poor support for her 15-stone husband, who will sink into it so that his wife is literally trying to sleep on the other side of a hill. Neither of them will rest properly.

Even so, the problem is not as insoluble as it appears, for most bedding manufacturers produce mattresses with several spring tensions to cater for varying weights. Double bed mattresses can now be bought with different spring tensions on each side — one for the lightweight wife, one for the heavyweight husband. Or vice versa. In some cases these mattresses actually consist of two single mattresses joined by a zip-fastener, which is almost unnoticeable so far as it affects comfort.

The subject of sleep is described, along with suggestions for mattresses, in a pamplet published by the Central Council for Health Education, Tavistock House, Tavistock Square, London, WC1.

TEETH
Abscess. This appears as a result of infection from a decayed tooth. Several varying conditions may arise depending on the situation and the course taken by the pus.

In most cases removal of the tooth is necessary. Certainly early dental treatment should be sought.

Dental Decay in Children. Care and treatment of teeth should start for children as soon as their teeth appear. The number of milk teeth is usually 20 and these begin to break through the gums at any time between the sixth and 30th month. The centre front teeth on the lower jaw appear first, followed by the corresponding upper teeth, and then the rest.

The enamel and dentine of teeth are the hard coverings of the teeth (enamel is the polished exterior, dentine the bony interior). The amounts of enamel and dentine vary in different people, and depend on:

1. The nature of the first teeth; 2. Subsequent care of the teeth; 3. Health of the individual; 4. The action of the saliva.

It is not difficult to ensure fine, healthy teeth, provided good attention is paid to their early development and care. Parents should adopt the following measures to ensure their children's teeth are healthy. The child should then adopt these habits automatically and continue them.

1. Chew thoroughly all food. Hard crusts and biscuits should be given to all babies and young children, followed by other hard foods which need lots of chewing. Biting on a plastic or bone teething ring is essential.

2. No food or sweets should be allowed between meals.

3. The mouth and teeth should be cleaned thoroughly *before a child goes to bed*, with a soft baby toothbrush and milk of magnesia. This time is more important than in the morning.

4. Particles of food should never be allowed to stay between the teeth.

5. After the age of three, it is essential for a child to have regular dental attention at not less than six-monthly intervals. This is imperative, whether or not there is any pain or decayed teeth.

Gingivitis. Inflammation of the gums which starts around the teeth and causes bleeding. As the condition develops, the inflamed gums swell and begin to draw away from the teeth. The gums are extremely sensitive and it is painful to chew.

One cause of gingivitis is failure to brush the teeth. Tiny particles of food lodge between the teeth, or between teeth and gums. This leads to gum infection. Other potential causes of gingivitis are tartar on the teeth, decaying teeth, and false teeth that produce gum irritation. Poor health and a poor diet may accelerate gingivitis.

If left untreated gingivitis can permanently damage the gums and cause loss of teeth. Good, regular dental care is essential. The dentist or hygienist will scale away the tartar, treat the decayed teeth, make certain fillings are in order, and false teeth fit correctly.

Ideally, brush the teeth — in upwards and downwards strokes in a circular movement — after every meal. And always immediately before going to bed and on getting up in the morning. Go light on sugary foods and maintain a well-balanced diet.

Gumboil. This is an abscess on the gum at the root of a decayed tooth. Pain can be relieved with an analgesic, the infection with antibiotics. When the swelling goes down, the patient should have the tooth treated by a dentist.

Pyorrhoea. A condition in which pus comes away from the teeth sockets and is accompanied by swollen and inflamed gums. As the infection persists the gums recede and the teeth may become loose.

Dental treatment is essential.

THE NATIONAL
HEALTH SERVICE

Most people make use of the National Health Service through their doctor, the dentist, chemist or optician. Perhaps even through medical or surgical treatment in hospital.

Every type of treatment — providing it is medically necessary and available — can be obtained on the National Health. This includes abortion and even cosmetic nose surgery.

Key figure in all this is your own local doctor, or general practitioner as he is sometimes called. Each patient must register on a doctor's list. The doctor gives all necessary treatment, though on certain occasions he may think a specialist's opinion advisable. It is through your doctor you go to hospital.

Ambulances. A doctor can call an ambulance as a free service to get to hospital a patient who is unfit to travel by public transport.

Changing your Doctor. If the patient moves home, even if it is only a few doors away in the same street, he at once has the right to choose a new doctor. All he needs to do is complete the appropriate space inside his medical card and present it to the new doctor.

If the patient has moved within the same district and chooses to stay on his own doctor's list, he must notify the Executive Council explaining the change of address. The Executive Council then issue a new medical card with the correct, up-to-date details. *The patient may not of his own accord change the address on the front of his own medical card.*

Sometimes a patient wants to change his doctor while he is still living at the same address. This can be done in two ways.

He can get his doctor's agreement to the change, and ask him to sign the appropriate space in the medical card. The patient then gives this card to his new doctor. Because of the obvious embarrassment this method is rarely used.

The usual way is by transfer slip. The patient sends the medical card to the Executive Council with a letter asking for a transfer slip to be stuck on the card so that he can change his doctor. The Executive Council sends back the card with a white sticker inside (the transfer slip). The patient fills this in with his name and address and presents it to the new doctor.

If the doctor accepts the patient, the doctor sends this card back to the Executive Council who then transfer the patient to the new doctor's list two weeks later. The patient gets a new medical card showing the transfer.

Chiropody. There is a shortage of chiropodists. However certain local authorities do provide a very good service for the elderly.

Dental Treatment. Schoolchildren can attend the dentist at the local health clinic if one is available. Both adults and children can go to any dentist who accepts NHS patients.

A patient who doesn't give his dentist enough notice that he cannot keep his appointment, enabling the dentist to book another patient, is liable to pay a fee. If the dentist cannot use the time for an alternative patient, he can charge the patient who doesn't turn up a fee.

For every NHS patient a fee up to a maximum of £10 is chargeable for a course of treatment. The exceptions are children, pregnant mothers and old age pensioners.

Dental treatment is free: for children under 16; older children still full-time at school; those between 16 and 21 who have left school (except for false teeth and alterations to teeth); expectant mothers and women who have had a baby in the previous 12 months.

The following persons and their dependents are also entitled to free dental treatment: those who are receiving supplementary benefit, family income supplement, and free medical prescriptions and free milk and vitamins because they are in the low income group.

The Doctor's Rights. A doctor has the right to refuse to accept any patient on his list — without explanation. He also has the right to rid himself of a patient by asking the

Executive Council to take the patient off his list. But if the patient needs medical treatment it is the doctor's duty to give this during the period the patient is finding a new doctor. *But it is the doctor who decides whether this treatment is necessary.*

The Executive Council send the patient a letter stating the date on which the doctor will have no more responsibility for him.

Emergencies. If there is a real medical emergency and the patient's own doctor isn't available, then the patient has the right to send for any nearby National Health doctor, to get that emergency treatment. This right should not be used too lightly, because if the case turns out to be just sheer panic the attending doctor might charge a fee.

Emergencies such as accidents in the home, poisoning, burns, etc., and all accidents or cases of sudden illness in the street entitle a patient to have an emergency ambulance called by a member of the public. This enables the patient to reach hospital without a doctor in attendance.

The emergency ambulance can be called by using any telephone and dialling the emergency number listed in the telephone box. Or by asking the telephone operator, if the phone is not on the dialling system.

Eye Treatment and Spectacles. If you want an eye test see your doctor, taking your medical card to the surgery, and you will be given an OSCI form. The patient takes this to an optician or medical ophthalmologist (many practise from an optician's premises), who will test the eyes and, if necessary, prescribe spectacles.

If an eye disease is discovered the optician reports back to the doctor so that you can go to an eye specialist.

Once a patient has his OSCI form he is entitled to visit the optician for an annual eye test without referring to his doctor.

Spectacles are free: for children under the age of 16 and for older children still full-time at school. Exempt from most charges are those on supplementary benefit, family income supplement, and people in the low income group who get a free medical prescription and free milk and vitamins.

Spectacle prescriptions are free: for children under 16; men of 65 and over, women of 60 and over; expectant mothers; the mother of a baby under 12 months; people suffering from specific medical conditions. Exemption certificates are issued to those on supplementary benefit, family income supplement, or who have a war or service disablement pension.

These free prescriptions also apply to elastic hosiery, supplied as medically necessary.

The Family Doctor Service. Certain rules do apply once a patient is registered on a doctor's list. If you're choosing a GP for the first time, friends or neighbours may recommend one in your area). You can get a list of local doctors from the National Health Service Executive Council, whose address is in your telephone directory under NHS. Lists are available too in main post offices, public libraries, and citizens' advice bureaux.

The patient must attend the doctor's surgery for advice and treatment unless he is too ill to do so. *Then* he is entitled to ask his doctor to call. When asking a doctor to visit you at home you must explain your reason, for it has been laid down officially that it is the doctor who must make this decision.

As contraception is now free for all women your doctor can provide this service. He may prescribe either *The Pill*, one of several variations of the *inter-uterine device* (known as the I.U.D.), the *Diaphragm* (Dutch Cap) or whatever he and his patient feel best suited to her both from a health and personal point of view.

Financial Hardship. Patients in need of financial help can apply to the local officer of the Department of Health and Social Security for supplementary benefit.

Home Helps. Any patient who for medical reasons is unable to cope with housework can get a certificate from her doctor stating what she needs and the reasons. This goes to the local public health clinic where arrangements can be made for a Home Help to attend *if one is available*. The Help will only attend for a set number of hours each day to do the heavy work and occasionally cook a meal. She is not in a position to stay all day with a patient as free companion and housekeeper.

Laundry. Those suffering from disorders which cause a lot of laundering of bed linen can be helped. The family doctor will assess the patient's need for laundry facilities and possibly incontinence pads, and contact either the local authority's social services department or the area health authority. If the patient is on supplementary benefit, it is possible to get an allowance to cover the cost of laundry and wear and tear on sheets.

Medical Certificates. During illness a patient has the right to get free certificates from the doctor so as to claim Sickness Benefit or Industrial Injury Benefit. He should send this certificate to the local National Insurance office within three days of being taken ill. If he delays he may lose the right to some of his sickness benefit. Alternatively he can send a private letter during those three days saying that a medical certificate will follow, registering the actual date of the start of his illness.

If on the initial visit the doctor knows his patient will be well enough to resume work seven days later, he can issue one 'first and final' certificate. Otherwise a patient must get certificates at intervals to cover the whole sickness period and *must not go back to work until the doctor has issued a final certificate.* If this last rule is broken the doctor is not allowed to give a final certificate and the patient may lose benefit.

During the period covered by these official certificates no insurance stamps must be fixed to the Insurance Card. So even if the patient doesn't want to claim sickness benefit — perhaps because he is self-employed or has his wages made up by his employer — he should still send in certificates to cover the illness period, or he may have to pay for unnecessary insurance stamps.

National Health certificates are issued free by the doctor for National Insurance purposes; this is the only reason for which they can be issued.

If a patient needs certificates simply to notify an employer or to claim private benefits from a sick club, then he must ask his doctor for a private certificate. For this the doctor will charge a fee.

Nursing. Patients who need limited nursing at home can be visited free by the District Nurse on doctor's orders.

Nursing Equipment. If this is needed for a patient at home it can be loaned free of charge, providing it is certified as necessary by the District Nurse or family doctor. The local Social Services welfare officer obtains these items from welfare or the Red Cross.

Old People — the Geriatric Service. When a person is unable to look after himself/herself through infirmity or old age the patient can be admitted to an old people's hospital or nursing home. Increasingly, the modern idea is to provide hostels to accommodate 20 to 40 people, provided by the local authority.

Elderly people who need medical treatment are admitted to an ordinary hospital where geriatric beds are set aside in special wards.

Registering on a Doctor's List. A patient is provided with a medical card and on the front of this is the doctor's name, the patient's National Health number, name and address. Also on the front is printed the name and address of the area Executive Council. A number of rules for patients are printed on the back. Inside the card it explains how to change your doctor if either the doctor or the patient wish to do this.

No doctor has to accept a patient on his list. If a patient finds it difficult to get on a doctor's list he should write and explain this to the area Executive Council, who will advise, and in the last resort has powers to allocate a patient to a doctor's list.

When a newborn baby has its birth registered the Registrar of Births hands the parent a card which should be completed and handed to the family doctor, so that the baby can be registered on the doctor's list.

A new arrival in Britain, and anyone who has never had a National Health Service doctor before, can call on a GP and fill up an application form. This will register him on that doctor's list and later a medical card will arrive through the post from the Local Executive Council.

Each family doctor has a self-imposed area in which he is willing to visit patients. If a patient moves out of this area he will have to register with a doctor in the new area.

A patient can only register on a doctor's list if he is going to stay in that area for at least three months. If staying for a shorter period he must register as a temporary patient (see below).

Special Equipment. There are over half a million handicapped people of all sorts — the deaf, dumb, blind, the physically deformed — in Britain.

If a person is crippled by a disease which prevents him travelling by public transport his doctor can send him to an orthopaedic surgeon for assessment. As a result, the Department of Health and Social Security may supply free either a mechanical chair or an invalid car.

From January 1, 1976, a new £5-a-week mobility allowance extended practical help to the most serious of all physically handicapped people — the 100,000 or so people who cannot walk. The recipients are able to use the money to aid themselves in any way they wish — to hire taxis, pay friends for driving them about, buy new shoes or go on holiday.

Some handicapped people qualify for the invalid car but not necessarily for the mobility allowance. No one is able to have the car and the allowance.

Claim forms for the mobility allowance, which is taxable, are available from the local office of the Department of Health and Social Security.

Temporary Patients. If the patient is away from home, whether on business or holiday, and needs medical attention, he can call on any doctor and register as a temporary patient. The doctor will give the patient a form to sign. This covers a temporary stay of up to three months. The patient must state whether he is in the area for more or less than 15 days.

Treatment under the NHS. A patient is entitled to any or all medical treatment necessary to diagnose his illness and for his recovery. This is at the sole discretion of the doctor.

If the local hospital cannot treat him, then he can be transferred to a hospital where he will get such specialist treatment. Any doctor will try to satisfy his patient by getting him into the hospital he prefers. But the doctor isn't bound to send his patient to any particular hospital, especially if it is too far away to be convenient.

The patient cannot insist on a certain surgeon performing

the operation. Though usually the surgeon who first sees the patient at his Out Patient clinic is the one who performs the operation.

Today the wide range of operations carried out include abortion, and sterilisation of both men and women — to prevent a couple having any more children. Vasectomy is the increasingly popular sterilisation operation for men. *However, these operations are only performed in some hospitals.*

When the family doctor treats a patient he gives him a prescription which any chemist in the country doing NHS dispensing will make up. In each area there is always one chemist open late on weekdays and for a brief period on Sunday mornings. Bank Holidays are the same as for Sundays.

Medicines and tablets left over after you have recovered from an illness should not be stored for the next time you're ill. Some medicines become useless, other disintegrate and can be dangerous. Eye-drops are a typical example.

Flush those left-over medicines down the toilet or get your doctor's advice about their disposal. Never put drugs in a dustbin, on a rubbish heap, or in any place where they can be found by children or animals.

COMMON ILLNESSES AND MEDICAL GUIDE

The object of this section is to outline everyday illnesses which affect us so that they can be more easily recognised, and to indicate what early precautions can be taken to ease the problem, and whether or not the doctor is needed urgently.

Abscess. These are painful, infected areas in which pus forms. They can occur in any part of the body, and may be either internal or external. A common site is the mouth, as a result of infected teeth, gums or tonsils, but they do soon spread to other parts of the body.

Symptoms initially may be abrupt, with sudden swelling and inflammation, as well as pain, due to poisons being absorbed into the system.

Most characteristic general signs are a rise of temperature, rapid pulse, and fits of shivering sometimes accompanied by vomiting.

Treatment by penicillin, or the sulpha group of drugs, may abort or localise an abscess quickly and prevent surgery. Consult a doctor early. Don't delay.

Adenoids. These small glands behind the point where the nose passages enter the back of the throat are usually associated with enlarged tonsils. Like the tonsils, their purpose is to block the entry of germs into the lungs and destroy them. Children are the usual victims of infected adenoids, but adults can be affected too.

Symptoms: Headache, bad breath, breathing through the mouth, dullness and an expressionless face, deafness often with discharge from the ears, snoring and sniffing of the nose due to catarrh, and a persistent cough at night when a child is lying flat. There is also a nasal tone to the voice.

Treatment: The symptoms of enlarged, infected adenoids

may be eased and the catarrhal discharge checked by spraying frequently with 1 per cent ephedrine in a normal saline solution. Asthma attacks and occasional bed-wetting may occur in someone with enlarged adenoids and 'pigeon' or 'barrel' chest result. An operation is the only cure. So the doctor should be consulted. Usually tonsils and adenoids are removed simultaneously. Afterwards, breathing exercises will be of great help.

Anaemia. A blood disorder in which the red cells are lower or have less haemoglobin (the pigment that gives red blood cells their colour) than normal. These cells play a vital role in breathing, because they carry oxygen inhaled into the lungs to all tissues of the body.

Anaemia may be a mild disorder because the person has too little iron in the system (as with a pregnant woman and older people); it may be due to a simple loss of blood by haemorrhage. But it is usually a symptom of some other disease. It develops in advanced stages of cancer and kidney failure.

Symptoms: Vary according to how severe it is. But the patient is unusually pale, particularly in the fingernails, lips, palms and lining of the eyelids. There may be an almost constant feeling of tiredness and a low temperature. In serious cases there may be dizziness, heart pounding, shortness of breath, and loss of appetite.

Treatment: See the doctor, who will diagnose from a blood test just how severe the problem is and give the necessary treatment.

Anoxeria Nervosa. In recent years, with the pressures to keep slim for fashion's sake, many adolescent girls have dieted themselves into this condition. The patient starts off 'just slimming' but begins to eat little or no food, for psychological reasons. Unless expert advice is sought, the severe wasting that results eventually leads to death.

On the other hand there is the person who eats too much. This can be a sign of physical disease, particularly when the victim loses weight sharply, but usually the compulsive eater (often a teenager or lonely older person) does it for emotional reasons to compensate for lack of love and attention.

Appendicitis *(acute)*. This common disease — inflammation of the appendix — may prove fatal if the signs and symptoms are misunderstood. It usually happens in childhood or adolescence, but can occur at any age.

Symptoms: If it starts suddenly, as in an acute case, the pain persists in the area of the navel, and soon moves to become a pain in the right side of the abdomen. It resembles a severe case of 'the stitch', so it is important it should not be mistaken for this relatively innocent and usually very temporary state. The pain is often followed by vomiting, a rise in temperature and a rapid pulse. Even when there is no change of temperature, but sudden acute pain in the right side in a child, followed by vomiting, send for a doctor.

Appendicitis *(chronic)*. This may be the sequel to an acute attack which has subsided or as a series of not so severe attacks.

There is constant pain and discomfort in the right side, often increased by exertion. Sometimes the symptoms are in the stomach or duodenum area and resemble a peptic ulcer.

Treatment: Whether it is an acute or chronic condition, see your doctor and arrange for an X-ray and other tests. Most often the doctor will diagnose appendicitis right away and arrange for an immediate operation.

Aspirin. A drug, prescribed mainly as a pain-killer, it is also useful in reducing fever and pain in arthritis. Properly used, it is effective and safe (one or two tablets every three or four hours for an adult, and never more than 12 tablets in a 24-hour period; small doses for children or children's aspirin).

No one who is prone to stomach or duodenal ulcers should take aspirin without consulting a doctor as it can induce bleeding. The usual alternative is Paracetamol.

Asthma. A disorder of the bronchial tubes, causing great difficulty in breathing. Most asthmatic attacks are mild but the condition is chronic and if it remains untreated can become serious. The two chief causes are an allergic reaction, which is usually inherited, and infection of the nose, sinuses and the bronchial tubes leading to the lungs, or of the lungs

45

themselves. In allergic asthma, the sufferer may be sensitive to pollen, animal hairs, house dust, insecticides, certain foods and drugs.

A nervous person or someone under emotional stress is far more likely to suffer frequent asthma attacks. Tiredness can trigger off a spasm of asthma, so can certain weather conditions.

Symptoms: The individual feels a tightness in his chest. He coughs, wheezes, and has difficulty in breathing. He may feel he is suffocating and his face may turn blue. It can be frightening but is not generally dangerous. Towards the end of an attack, the victim coughs up thick mucus, which gives him some relief.

Treatment: Infection can be controlled by antibiotics, and a doctor may prescribe a series of injections to reduce the victim's sensitivity.

Asthma sufferers can control their condition by using an inhaler containing adrenaline or salbutamol. The doctor may inject hydrocortisone into a vein in severe cases, and prescribe further treatment.

There are several ways an asthmatic can help himself and minimise the effects of his condition — by looking after his general health, by avoiding constipation, flatulence and gastro-intestinal disturbances, by seeking medical treatment immediately for nasal obstruction or bronchitis, by never eating a heavy meal late at night, by practising deep breathing exercises, and by living in a warm, dry area rather than a damp one.

Attendance at a clinic for skin tests and vaccine treatment is advised for anyone suffering from asthma.

Athlete's Foot. Excessive perspiration aggravates this chronic infection of the skin between the toes. It is caused by a fungus that thrives in wet, warm places like swimming pools, which is where it is often picked up.

Symptoms: Splits in the skin, blisters and scaling between the toes, and sometimes on the sole of the foot. The fungus can also produce an unpleasant smell.

Treatment: With a minor infection rub away the scales, dry the foot and apply a little rubbing alcohol. Dry again and dust with a mild deodorant powder. The more the foot is exposed to the fresh air at this stage the better. Before going to bed and first thing in the morning, a mild fungicidal cream should be applied.

A footbath in potassium permanganate solution, as advised by the doctor, will soothe and cure oozing blisters. The feet should be soaked for 15 minutes, dried, and calamine lotion applied.

Clean socks each day (cotton or wool which absorb sweat, rather than nylon which doesn't) are vital. And light shoes. If the infection continues consult a doctor.

Autism. The state of living in a fantasy world as a means of escape from the real world. Autism often shows itself in childhood. The autistic child is completely absorbed in himself. He doesn't relate to people, appears insensitive to pain and, if anyone speaks to him, doesn't show the slightest response.

Symptoms: An early warning is when a child doesn't answer his parents when they speak, doesn't smile or respond to them, and they can't get through to him. His line of communication is limited to a few signs and signals. The autistic child can get unusually attached to a toy or some other object. Sometimes he is full of activity, at others totally withdrawn.

Treatment: Psychological and occupational therapy at a special centre or school. Tranquillising drugs can be of some help.

Anyone with a child suffering from autism may find guidance from the National Society for Autistic Children, 1, Golders Green Road, London, NW11.

Backache. Pain in the back can be a symptom of various abnormal conditions of the body. Kidney disease or gall bladder infection; constipation, pregnancy, prolapse of the womb; pneumonia or influenza; severe menstrual disorder. Or the pain may involve the back itself, a strain, bad posture, or slipped disc can cause backache.

Women often suffer from backache and if it arises through pregnancy or difficult periods, then it is an abnormal feature of these conditions and the patient should have medical advice.

Disorders of the spinal muscles. Into this category come all forms of muscular rheumatism, lumbago, and fibrositis, which are generally due to exposure to cold and damp.

Over-tiredness, bad posture, a job which means prolonged stooping and unnecessary bending of the spine — like typing at a desk the wrong height — all contribute to these conditions. The result, severe pain in the spinal muscles.

Treatment for a strained back is a few days in bed, preferably on a firm mattress. Heat from a hot water bottle or electric blanket may ease the pain. Afterwards, careful exercise and physiotherapy restores the correct movement and prevents continued backache.

Lumbago is a sudden pain in the back, especially after a game of football or òutdoor exercise, or standing in a draught. A man can find himself unable to stand up straight or even move at all. Usually there is one tender spot in the back muscles, which are in spasm.

Treatment: A mild case generally recovers in a few days, but a doctor may inject pain-killing drugs to ease the pain in the meantime.

Diseases of the spinal column. These are far more serious, demanding the specialised skill of an orthopaedic surgeon, as the pain in the back is caused by diseased joints which may need surgical skill or manipulation.

Nervous backache *can* happen when there is nothing really wrong with the person except their state of mind and instability.

Treatment: This will depend on the doctor's diagnosis of the patient's general condition or the specific disease from which he is suffering. If the condition cannot be put right surgically the doctor will rely mainly on correcting the diet, supplying the necessary vitamins, massage and special treatment, surgical belts, etc., according to the nature and site of the pain.

Slipped Discs. This is when the 'shock absorber' gristle discs between two of the spine's vertebrae move out of place, wear away, split or grind against each other and press against the spinal nerves. Often the sufferer remembers his back 'going' as he picked up a heavy weight. If the discs press on his sciatic nerve, the sciatic pain shoots down his back and legs. Otherwise he gets lumbago, radiating down both legs with a numbness and tingling in the legs or feet.

Treatment: Consult an orthopaedic surgeon, who will X-ray the spine and establish that two of the vertebrae are riding close together, indicating the disc has collapsed. He will prescribe physiotherapy, special exercises, a surgical belt. Occasionally, an operation may be performed.

A similar condition, which used to be called osteo-arthritis of the neck spinal joints has a new name, spondylosis. The neck joints show on X-ray that they are worn away.

Symptoms are neck pains, sometimes travelling right up and over the skull, and stiffness in moving the neck.

Treatment: A felt collar, neck supports, physiotherapy, according to what the specialist thinks best.

Bad Breath *(Halitosis).* A bad breath isn't the one that smells of garlic or onions after a particularly spicy meal. True halitosis is the result of decayed teeth, diseased gums, tonsils, nose, lungs or sinuses. Many other conditions cause it, including disorders of the stomach and intestines, or blood poisoned by urinary wastage.

Treatment: Brush the teeth regularly, morning and night, and after each meal. Consult the dentist twice a year, whether your breath is bad or not. Gargles and mouthwashes may mask bad breath temporarily, but if it persists, see your doctor.

Bed Sores *(Decubitus Ulcer).* A serious condition, the result of lying in bed in one position during illness. Most susceptible are the elderly, the bedridden with nervous and circulation complaints, and those for whom paralysis makes a change of position impossible.

Neglect and bad nursing can accelerate bed sores. But in cases of prolonged illness of the bedridden, in diseases associated with wasting, and where there is chronic pus discharge, a bed sore may be difficult to prevent.

When a person lies down the bulk of the body bears down on a few small areas. It is to these areas, in someone sick, that the blood supply to the soft tissues of the skin is reduced. A healthy person can turn over and relieve the pressure. Someone sick, in serious pain or too weak to move, will get a breakdown of the tissues. Small red patches on the skin are the first signs. If neglected, these become hard and blue and develop into ulcers.

Bed sores are easier to prevent than to heal. If the patient cannot change his own position in bed, he should be helped — *this is very important*. Air cushions, water

49

cushions, and in some cases a water bed, will help prevent bed sores. Or, if formed, they will prevent pain.

It is vital that the patient's skin is kept clean and healthy by frequent bed baths and massage. The bed sheets should be smoothed down often to remove creases and crumbs. The patient should be washed and dried in stages. First, wash the lower part of the back and the bottom with soap and water. Dry thoroughly, then bathe with surgical spirit or eau-de-Cologne, followed by an antiseptic.

It is essential that excretions are removed in the prevention of bed sores. Particularly in patients suffering from urine incontinence or convalescing at home after a bladder operation, when the wound is still leaking.

If the skin has become red or broken before an ulcer has occured, strapping the affected area with Elastoplast is a useful way of preventing the sore developing. The following treatment will be necessary if the ulcer has developed:

Treatment: Apply the BPC ointment of Balsam of Peru, or a cream of zinc, castor oil and Friar's Balsam to help healing. The ulcer should be kept clean with compresses of warm normal saline. Healing will be hastened if this is followed by applying gauze soaked in penicillin lotion made with normal saline. This treatment must always be administered after advice from a doctor and his prescription.

In intractable bed sores, where all treatment has failed, an Elastoplast strapping may succeed.

Bed Wetting *(Enuresis).* Many children cannot overcome the habit of wetting the bed until their bladders have grown enough to hold a night's production of urine (just over half a pint). They do so usually by four or five. When a child is ready, both emotionally and physically, he learns control. A parent shouldn't be over-anxious.

Bed wetting seems to run in families. Continued enuresis is often due to emotional insecurity. Perhaps a child feels shut out with the arrival of a new baby, or there is sickness in the family, or the parents have parted.

There are various ploys which sometimes work. One is to restrict refreshments for two hours before bedtime, without making a fuss about it. The child should be reminded to go to the toilet before going to bed. Some parents get good results by waking the child gently at about 11.0 p.m.

and taking him to the toilet in his drowsiness. Never scold or punish, but it is a good idea to praise a child on his 'dry' nights.

Blood Transfusion. Modern surgery is only possible because of the availability of blood for transfusion. Some operations can only be done with the ready availability of eight pints of blood from the Blood Bank.

Anybody willing to give a pint of blood can find the address of the nearest Blood Bank by looking in the local telephone directory.

Boil *(Furuncle).* An inflated, tender, pus-filled area on the skin caused by a bacterial infection, usually Staphylococcus Aureus. The bacteria enter the skin through a hair follicle, sweat gland, scratch or other broken spot. Sometimes sweating or dirt precipitates infection. To avoid boils, keep clean and try to prevent friction — such as too-tight collars — where sweat may collect. The back of the neck is often susceptible to boils for this reason. A boil may occur if someone is run down in health, anaemic or whose resistance is lowered by a poor diet. It is sometimes a complication of acne in adolescents.

Treatment: Antibiotics. An antiseptic should be painted around the boil to prevent the infection spreading. An Elastoplast strapped over the boil will bring it to a head more quickly. A kaolin poultice will bring a boil to a head and cause pus to discharge.

If it has to be incised, this should be left to a doctor, particularly in the case of children or old people, and where there are several boils or one large painful one. After the boil bursts magnesium sulphate paste should be applied and protected with lint or Elastoplast with a small hole cut in the centre to allow the discharge to escape. Fucidin ointment applied every four hours will soon clear it up. If the boils are widespread, a daily bath with some antiseptic in the water is essential.

Check that you are taking the right balance of vitamins and that your diet is a healthy one.

Where boils recur, consult your doctor, who will probably examine the urine to see if there is sugar and albumin (possibly indicating diabetes or kidney trouble).

Breast *(Inspection of)*. Checking the breasts is a simple precaution *every* woman between 18 and 60 should take once a month throughout her life.

This 'early warning' drill is a guard against breast cancer, which kills more than 12,000 women a year in Britain.

A lump in the breast is usually a harmless cyst or nodule and not necessarily a symptom of cancer. But it *can* be — and the earlier a lump is found and diagnosed by a doctor and/or specialist, the greater the chance of a complete cure.

The following do-it-yourself test should be made just after a woman's monthly period ends, if she is still menstruating:

Sit in front of the bedroom mirror and study your breasts for the following: a change in their appearance or shape, inverted nipples, bleeding or discharge from the nipples, a small tuck or crease you haven't noticed before. Then lie on your back and examine each breast. You will be more comfortable if you lie on a pillow:

1. With the flats of the fingers examine the tissues under the armpit.

2. Feel the upper, outer quarter of the breast. This area needs special attention.

3. Next, check the rest of the outer half of the breast by moving the fingers round the edge to the area at the centre near the nipple.

4. Press the inner half of the breast against the wall of the chest, moving the fingers from the breastbone to the middle of the breast around the nipple.

5. Feel the nipple area, then the rest of the inner half of the breast. Place the pillow or pad under the other shoulder and examine the other breast.

Remember, if there *is* anything unusual, see your doctor *immediately*.

Bronchitis. This, strictly speaking, is inflammation of the bronchial tubes. Mild cases may seem like a severe chest cold. In its worst form it may lead to pneumonia.

Bronchitis, sometimes called the 'English disease', causes more than 30,000 deaths every year in Britain. The young and the old are most often struck down, and in these cases it can become more serious.

Acute bronchitis: This is often due to a virus, such as

a cold or influenza. But sometimes it is linked to measles, chicken-pox, whooping cough, an allergy, or chemical irritants such as ammonia fumes.

Symptoms: A cold with a headache behind the eyes, sore throat, fullness in the head, back pain and aching joints, and a general ill feeling. There may be a rise in temperature and some people feel sick. To start with the cough is often dry and painful, and there is a tight feeling in the chest. Later, the cough loosens and the sufferer may start breathing rather quickly. Acute bronchitis often occurs in bad weather and may recur in a susceptible person. It usually lasts 10 days to two weeks.

Treatment: Send for the doctor early. Meantime, inhaling one teaspoonful of Friar's Balsam in a pint of boiling water three times a day will bring relief. A simple linctus will help ease the cough. Then it is up to the doctor.

Chronic bronchitis: Patients who really are subject to recurring attacks of bronchitis should see their doctor *before* early autumn, as there are vaccine injections which can keep bronchitis at bay.

Bronchitis in its most chronic form may follow repeated chest infections, or be a reaction to excessive smoking. It is very common in industrial areas and strikes more men than women. Skilled medical advice is necessary, as a chest X-ray may be needed.

Bunion *(Hallux Valgus)*. This is a painfully deformed big toe, usually the result of wearing badly fitting, too tight shoes that push it in towards the other toes. This puts pressure on the joint connecting it with the foot. Continued irritation causes a bony deposit and a pouch of tissues forms over it. An inflamed bunion may develop into arthritis of the joint.

Bunions can be avoided by wearing correctly fitting shoes from an early age. Slight pain can be relieved by resting the foot on a hot water bottle but a chiropodist should be consulted for corrective treatment. Surgery is occasionally required.

Carbuncle. Perhaps the first sign of diabetes, which is why in all cases the urine should be examined by a doctor.

A carbuncle is larger and goes deeper into the skin than a boil, which it resembles, and tends to spread to other parts of the body. Like a boil, it is an eruption of the skin with a hard surface and is filled with pus. It is most often found where there are sweat glands or hair — on the chest, neck, face, between the thighs and under the arms.

Treatment: The same as for boils, with the addition of penicillin or Sulphadiazin injections, or other antibiotics. Sometimes, if the carbuncle is big, it may require a free surgical operation under local anaesthetic.

Cervical Smear. A quick and simple early warning method of detecting, or preventing cancer of the neck of the womb.

The cyto test, as it is sometimes called, takes three minutes and picks up any abnormalities in the structure of the cells that might develop into cancer as far ahead as 10 to 15 years. Most often it is other very minor conditions that are discovered.

Between three and five women in every 1,000 have a positive result. What happens then is a simple operation, called a cone biopsy, in which a finger-nail sized piece of tissue is removed. This involves a couple of days in hospital.

Every woman from the age of sexual maturity should have the test at least every three years. Certainly if she is over 35, or has had three pregnancies.

Any woman who has difficulty in getting the test should contact the Women's National Cancer Control Campaign, 9, King Street, London, WC2.

Chicken-pox. A mild, feverish and infectious disease due to a virus, common among children.

Symptoms: The child usually feels unwell for 24 hours before the appearance of small red, raised spots on the scalp, neck, back, chest and shoulders, or on some of these parts of the body, but rarely on the face. The pimples dry up and drop off at about the fifth day, leaving very little of the pitting or scarring which follow smallpox. It is not a dangerous disease, the fever being neither very high nor lasting, but it is infectious for about 14 days after the appearance of the first symptoms.

Treatment: Send for the doctor. Keep the child in bed for a day or two and thereafter away from other children until the risk of spreading the infection has passed.

The virus of chicken-pox is related to that of shingles

and those in contact with a case of chicken-pox sometimes develop shingles. (See under Herpes).

Choking. Obstruction of the voice box or wind-pipe, which makes breathing difficult or impossible.

Call the doctor quickly, if there is a sudden obstruction. Then a hard slap between the shoulder blades or, in the case of a child, turn him upside-down without delay. There is no time to wait for a doctor. Anything that cuts off the oxygen supply is very dangerous.

Codeine. A pain-relieving drug, chemically similar to morphine. It can also control coughing. It is usually prescribed for pain more severe than can be dealt with by milder pain-killers.

Codeine may cause constipation, nausea and side effects in some people. Drowsiness and reduced reflex action are usual.

Dentists may prescribe it for patients who have lots of dental treatment.

Colic. Babies often experience this severe, spasmodic pain in the abdomen. In babies it is often the result of swallowing air during feeding, which is why they should be burped now and again. The baby's abdomen may be distended and as he cries he draws his legs up, releasing wind.

Treatment: Babies will find relief if hot (not too hot) poultices are placed on the abdomen. A half teaspoonful each of peppermint water and dill water in a little water will soothe the infant by dispersing the wind.

In adults colic may be caused by constipation, disorders of the intestines (such as gastro-enteritis), gall bladder or kidney (due to stones).

Treatment: Adults may also benefit from applying hot water to the abdomen. But it is vital that a correct diagnosis is made by a doctor, who will prescribe the appropriate treatment.

Common Cold. Many viruses, old and new, cause colds — infection of the lungs, particularly the nose, throat and bronchial tubes.

Symptoms: Stuffy or running nose, headache and cough, a feeling of chilliness, a reduction in the sense of smell and taste, listlessness, a slight fever. A sore throat and cough may follow.

Treatment: Rest in bed, isolate yourself. Take two aspirins every four hours if there is a fever, headache or sore throat. Or alternatively, Veganin or Dover's Powders. Lots of fluids and a light diet are recommended, especially where there is a fever. There are lots of remedies to make breathing easier, such as inhaling menthol, eucalyptus and Friar's Balsam, or nose douches.

Inoculations against colds can be effective in susceptible people from the early autumn. Lots of Vitamin C (particularly in oranges) should be taken as a defence against colds. Iron tonics and halibut-liver oil capsules are very helpful in restoring the appetite and overcoming weakness following a cold.

Constipation. Difficulty in emptying the bowel. Usually the waste material has become hard and compact, making it painful to expel.

Poor diet, nervous tension, insufficient exercise and routine use of laxatives may all contribute to this condition. Regular habits do not preclude the possibility of constipation. For incomplete elimination, despite regularity, may only load the lower bowel.

Symptoms: Many and varied — a general not-very-well feeling, lack of concentration, depression, headache, sleeplessness. The complexion may be muddy, the tongue furred, appetite poor and the breath unpleasant.

Straining in constipation may cause piles.

One bowel movement every 24 hours is average for most people. However, there are perfectly healthy people who go 36 or 48 hours, or even more, by habit, and do not suffer constipation.

If constipation is continuous, see a doctor. It is rarely serious, unless it is the result of an organic disease.

Contraception. Prevention of conception, or pregnancy, by various contraceptive devices. These include:

The Pill: Female sex hormone tablets taken on a regular monthly schedule, usually every day for 21 days, beginning on the fifth day after the start of menstruation.

This is the most reliable of all modern contraceptives, but a woman should discuss it with her doctor, as there are various types and strengths of The Pill. A woman may have to experiment before she finds one to suit her. Or she may not be medically fit enough to go on it. Side effects can include nausea, cramp, weight gain, and possible risk in certain women of a thrombosis.

Diaphragm (Dutch Cap): A dome-shaped rubber cap which fits over the mouth of the womb and prevents sperm from entering. A contraceptive foam or jelly is an added protection. The cap should be inserted before love-making and should stay in place at least eight hours afterwards. Initially, it should be fitted by a doctor or at a birth control clinic. It is about 88 per cent reliable, slightly less so than The Pill.

Intra-Uterine Device (I.U.D.): After sterilisation and The Pill, the most reliable method (about 97 per cent safe) of contraception.

The I.U.D. is a small piece of foreign material placed in the womb to prevent conception. Most common types are coils or loops of flexible plastic that can be easily inserted (by a doctor or at a birth control clinic) without stretching the neck of the womb. A small extension of the I.U.D. is usually left to protrude into the vagina, so that it is easy to remove. It also reassures a woman that she hasn't accidentally lost it.

The device can be left in position indefinitely, providing a check-up is made every two years.

A doctor doesn't normally fit an I.U.D. into a woman who hasn't had children. Some women cannot wear the I.U.D. because of persistent discomfort, the possibility of infection setting in, or because they keep on expelling it.

The Condom: Still the most commonly used form of contraception. This thin rubber sheath worn over the penis is highly reliable (86 per cent safe) if it is of good quality. A big advantage is that it offers some measure of protection against veneral disease.

Rhythm Method: So-called natural method of birth control, based on abstaining from sex during 10 days of each menstrual cycle. This covers the period when a woman ovulates and is therefore at her most fertile.

First, a woman must keep a daily record of her temperature for several months (the body temperature rises at the start of ovulation). She must allow for uncertainties by lengthening the period of abstinence and shortening the 'safe period'. In practice, she should not have sex from 10 days after the start of her period until another 10 days have elapsed.

This is a rather unreliable method and should not be risked if a woman's periods are in any way irregular.

Coitus Interruptus: Withdrawal of the penis from the vagina *before* sperm is ejaculated is still widely practised. This is the most risky method of birth control (barely 80 per cent effective). Also it is mentally frustrating for one or both partners, giving little satisfaction from the act of love.

Other Methods: Now in the experimental by trial stage are 'morning after' pills, taken the morning after intercourse; hormone injections given once every four to six months. Both are for women. A hormone contraceptive taken by men is also being tested.

Sterilisation: The ultimate method of birth control. It means no more children, no turning the clock back.

In recent years, with population pressures and a desire by many couples to restrict their family for all time, sterilisation has become much more acceptable. It is, except in rare almost freak cases, irreversable.

For a man it involves the increasingly popular minor operation, vasectomy, in which the sperm tubes leading from the testicles to the penis are either tied or, more usually, cut. For a woman, it means the slightly bigger operation of tying or severing the Fallopian Tubes, which carry the egg cells from the ovaries to the womb.

Corn. A type of callus, or thickening of the skin which appears on or between the toes. Almost always the result of pressure from very tight or badly fitting shoes.

Hard corns: These usually crop up where the skin or tissue over the bone is very thin.

Treatment: Home treatment with a razor blade may be the quick, obvious way to deal with it but, unless the root is removed, the corn will certainly recur. Meantime, there is the danger of infection and bleeding, and a worsening of the corn. A diabetic should *never* cut his or her own corns.

If only home treatment is possible, a collodion dressing is advised. But best to consult a expert chiropodist.

Soft corns: These occur between the toes, often because the area between the toes repeatedly hasn't been dried after a bath. And also through pressure.

Treatment: Separate the toes with felt or foam pads and dust night and morning with a powder of equal parts of starch, zinc oxide and alum.

Bathing the feet at night will harden soft or tender feet which perspire and tend to blister. Use normal saline and after drying carefully, rub with surgical or methylated spirit to which is added distilled extract of witch hazel. Or bathe in a weak solution of permanganate of potash, then dry and dust with one of the above powders.

With perspiring feet which tend to smell bathe in a weak solution of Dettol or Sanitas. Then dust between the toes and in the socks with one of the above powders. Wash the feet frequently and use a deodorant spray as and when necessary.

Cough. A protective reflex in which the windpipe or bronchial tubes try to get rid of whatever is blocking or irritating them. This is usually mucus from the nose or lungs which irritates the windpipe, and results in coughing. A cough *isn't* normal. Many people will ignore one which may last for years. This is dangerous, as a cough may be the sign of a far more serious disease.

A short dry cough, when nothing is brought up, may be the result of simply going out into the cold. Such a cough often accompanies an inflamed throat, tonsils or windpipe.

Coughing and a simultaneous sharp pain in the side could be a sign of pleurisy (inflamed outer linings of the lungs). Antibiotics and bed are what the doctor will order.

A barking cough which won't stop may indicate an enlarged heart, swollen glands in the chest, or a tumour of the lung or gullet. It may be a habit spasm which is called a nervous cough.

When phlegm isn't coughed up, then the cough may indicate tuberculosis in an older person or whooping cough in a child.

The cough that does bring up a lot of phlegm is usually due to too much smoking, bronchitis, chronic catarrh or sinusitis. A smoker's cough is at its worst in the mornings.

When children cough it usually means an infection of the lungs or bronchial tubes. But it can be caused by whooping cough, swollen tonsils, adenoids, a foreign body in the ear, nose or throat, a throat abscess or worms.

Nervous children — and those going through puberty — may have a cough with no physical basis.

Croup. An acute infection of the lungs and respiratory system, with easily identified symptoms — a hoarse, rasping voice and a cough like a barking seal.

Croup is most common in children and usually first crops up in the night. The cause can be germs or a virus infection. Someone with croup is often prone to allergies of various sorts. It can be dangerous, with difficulty in breathing, a fever, phlegm clogging the throat and windpipe, and in severe cases, blue lips.

Don't delay calling the doctor right away.

Curvature of the Spine. Muscular weakness of the back, which leads to overstraining the spine ligaments; physical deformity; rickets; stiff neck; bad posture through habit or a particular job. All these can cause this sad, unsightly condition.

Girls who have grown too quickly and are physically below par tend to get it. So do tall girls with long backs and muscles so weak they haven't the strength to exercise, and hold themselves straight. Round shoulders are the first sign, then some spinal curvature.

People who contract polio where one leg is wasted and shorter then the other, are often victims.

Treatment: The cause must be investigated first. Physical instruction with Swedish remedial exercises can improve the physique.

It is the duty of parents and teachers at school who notice children slouching or stooping to warn, and try to correct bad posture. Exercises and massage are vital in such children.

Cystitis. Infection and inflammation of the bladder. There is a frequent urge to pass urine, and when doing so a painful, burning sensation and sometimes bleeding. Fever, back and muscle pain, and vomiting may accompany an attack.

Cystitis affects four out of five women at some time in their lives, especially those who are sexually active, pregnant or past the menopause. It often subsides only to flare up again.

Hormone changes in the body, perhaps due to strain

and stress at childbirth or during the menopause, can cause it. So can too much love-making in certain women, thrush (a fungus-like infection of the vagina), and even antibiotics prescribed for women's internal infections. Tight nylon panties, use of strong detergents and washing powders, vaginal deodorants, highly scented soaps, skin sensitivity, careless washing and poor hygiene, and mystery viruses are also common causes.

Other contributory factors can be prolonged illness which lowers the body's resistance, renal and bladder disorders, diabetes, prolapse of the womb, bladder or vagina, and cancer.

Treatment: Fastidious care of the genitals to prevent further infection, a course of antibiotics (if suitable) or sulphonamides usually bring it under control. Sedatives may be necessary. Highly seasoned food, alcohol and anything that irritates the system should be avoided. If the condition persists, consult a doctor. The possibility of an X-ray may be explored.

Information and advice for mild or chronic sufferers can be obtained from Mrs Angela Kilmartin, U and I Club (Urinary Infection), 22 Gerrard Road, London N1.

Diarrhoea. Perpetual and excessive discharge of watery motions from the bowel. The entire system is debilitated, but the big danger is dehydration, as so much water is lost. Nourishment is affected because food passes through the intestines so quickly it can't be properly digested and absorbed into the system.

Diarrhoea has many causes. A mild attack can be precipitated by unwise eating and drinking. Some people are sensitive to certain foods — for example mussels, mushrooms, raw cabbage — and learn by experience that they cannot eat them without getting diarrhoea. Food poisoning causes more drastic attacks. There is usually nausea, vomiting and cramp. Poisons such as arsenic or lead also bring on severe reaction.

People who stay in one place develop a certain immunity to local conditions. Which is why foreign travel, especially to off-beat, poorer areas in hot weather, can cause diarrhoea, or what has commonly become known as 'Spanish tummy'. This is because of the change in water and diet, or of taking too much alcohol while travelling.

All holidaymakers should remember to drink only bottled or boiled water; to go easy on alcohol; to eat fresh fruit and vegetables only if cleaned and peeled; to avoid greasy food.

Treatment: Restore the body's fluid balance by drinking lots of liquids, such as tea, and thin soups. Kaolin is a good remedy available from the chemist, and *natural* yoghurt for a mildly upset tummy soon puts it right.

If diarrhoea lasts more than two days, see a doctor.

Dyslexia. Word blindness. Not just a question of being slow at reading, this is when a child is unable to read properly because the brain cannot sort out various letters.

Dyslexia doesn't indicate stupidity. In fact, some dyslexic children are very bright and above average intelligence.

The parent who spots this condition early enough can get advice about education from one of several dyslexia associations in this country.

Dyspepsia. Minor digestive disorder. But it should always be investigated as it can mask major and more serious diseases. The following symptoms should disappear quickly. If they don't, then do not hestitate to get a doctor's advice.

Symptoms: A feeling of fullness, which may vary from slight discomfort to some pain after meals, a burning sensation after food, with flatulence (due to gas in the stomach), a bitter taste in the throat because of acidity, and occasionally nervous vomiting. This is more prevalent in women.

A sallow, muddy complexion, furry tongue, bad taste in the mouth, constipation, mental depression, irritability and morning headaches may be linked with the above symptoms.

Treatment: Consult a doctor for an early, accurate diagnosis as to the cause of dyspepsia, and for immediate treatment for relief. An X-ray examination will exclude the possibility of a peptic ulcer, diseased or inflamed gall bladder, or a chronically inflamed appendix.

Embolism. This is blockage of blood vessels by either a blood clot, a fat globule, air, or bacteria. The material is carried through the blood and stops at a place too narrow for it to pass. There it stays.

A stroke is one result of an embolism. In this case the blood clot lodges in the brain or the neck, cutting off the blood supply to the brain which, starved, dies. The victim may lose his power of speech, the use of his limbs, and be unable to co-ordinate his movements.

Clots sometimes form in the legs (phlebitis) or obstruct an artery leading to an arm or leg, perhaps causing gangrene.

Treatment: Basically, the use of anti-coagulant drugs, which counteract the blood's tendency to clot; drugs to dilate the blood vessels, which help increase the flow of blood to nearby areas.

When there is a life-threatening embolism in, say, the lungs, surgery is necessary.

Flat Feet. This is when the entire sole of the foot rests flat on the ground, because the arch of the instep is lower than normal. It is sometimes hereditary. But may be due to long standing without good foot support, over-tiredness, over-weight, generally poor health following rickets, rheumatism, fever or any prolonged illness.

If one foot is affected more than the other in children, there may be curvature of the spine.

The condition means that the main bone of the foot is forced down, the muscle weakens and the instep disappears. The whole sole of the foot is lengthened and a normal walk becomes a sort of shuffle.

Treatment: Rest, massage and exercises, and particularly standing on the tips of the toes are a good idea early on. Skipping and running on the toes helps strengthen the feet. Walking on the edge of the foot with the toes turned in is another useful exercise later on. A dcotor may prescribe an arch support.

Children's feet should be examined regularly to see if they are flattening. Good posture is important to avoid flat feet.

Flatulence. Accumulation of air or wind in the stomach or intestines. Discomfort is relieved when the excess gas is passed out through the mouth or the back passage.

Most usual cause is the nervous habit of swallowing air. Belching may increase this if, as often happens, air is swallowed in the process of belching. Swallowing air is a symptom of anxiety and tension. Fizzy drinks also cause flatulence, so does eating gas-producing foods like onions, peas, cabbage, cucumber, fried foods, nuts, spices. These should be avoided by anyone with a tendency to flatulence.

Fluoride. A compound of the chemical, fluorine, and sodium or potassium. Tin and fluorine are an ingredient of several toothpastes and help prevent tooth decay.

Fluoride is also added to water in many cities and towns in Europe and North America.

Food Poisining. An acute illness resulting from eating contaminated food.

In rare cases poisons in food, such as shellfish, may affect the central nervous system and the victim's vision becomes blurred and his walk unsteady.

Most common food infection is salmonelosis. This can be picked up from shellfish growing in sewage-polluted water or from vegetables ' fertilised by human manure. Certain bacteria cause food to spoil. The most common is staphylococci. This contamination may happen when food is being handled or if it is kept in a warm room. Another bacteria surfaces in reheated cooked meat, producing colic and diarrhoea which sometimes resembles cholera. It can be fatal. If already cooked meat has to be reheated, do it slowly and thoroughly. Preferably never reheat pork.

Acute and chronic poisoning can develop from eating poisonous toadstools, plants or berries mistakenly thought to be edible, or from the residue of insecticides sprayed on fruit and vegetables.

Symptoms: These usually develop soon after the food is eaten but it can be 24 hours before the effects are felt. There is usually vomiting, diarrhoea, headache and a rash of varying intensity.

Treatment: Drink plenty of water to replace the body fluid lost in diarrhoea and vomiting.

A mild case of food poisoning may be over in a couple of days. But consult a doctor, who will prescribe the appropriate drugs if food poisoning is suspected.

Gargling. To relieve a mild sore throat, gargle every few hours with half a glass of warm water containing two crushed, or soluble, aspirin tablets. Then swallow it. Another useful gargle mixture is half a teaspoonful of salt in a large glass of warm water.

Call a doctor if you have a severe sore throat.

Gastro-Enteritis. Inflammation of the stomach and intestines. Most common causes are a contagious disease, an allergy, emotional upset, irritation of the intestine because of too much food or alcohol, or a drug or poison.

Symptoms: Fever, vomiting, diarrhoea. The consequent loss of fluids (dehydration) can be very serious, even fatal in a baby.

Treatment: Medicine such as kaolin-morphine will relieve the diarrhoea. Best to see a doctor. In the case of a baby, a doctor should be called immediately.

Giddiness. True giddiness (vertigo) is the feeling the world is spinning around and around, like riding on a whirling roundabout or looking down from a great height.

The cause is a disturbance of the fluid in the balancing mechanism of the inner ear, or it may be a sign of an ear or nerve disorder.

Dizziness is also the sensation that precedes fainting, when the brain is starved of blood or oxygen. Sometimes it is a sign of serious disease in the young. Though usually it is connected with emotional stress, hunger, early efforts at smoking, or travel sickness. Persistent giddiness, particularly in middle age, should be reported to a doctor.

Gout *(Podagra).* Abnormal amounts of uric acid (a breakdown product of proteins) upset the normal chemical processes of the body.

The result is a stiffening of joints of the body because the acid deposits have crystallised in the tissues. Sometimes the ears and kidneys are directly affected.

This disease most often strikes men over 30 and women after the menopause, though it is considerably rarer in women.

The exact reason for an attack isn't really known, except that it occurs when the level of uric acid in the blood is altered. Possible causes include: an accident, a surgical operation, a sudden change to a diet exceptionally rich in proteins and fat, such as liver and kidneys, taking medicines, or damage to an already affected joint. Often it is the big toe, only, that is affected in an acute attack of gout. It becomes hot, swollen, tender and very red.

Treatment: Anti-inflammatory drugs or steroids can usually relieve the pain within a few hours. Acute gout responds to a drug, colchicum, extracted from the autumn crocus. Long-term therapy with drugs to reduce the uric acid level is the main object of modern treatment.

Growing Pains. Not a normal symptom of growing up, though many parents seem to think so. Muscular pain in children is merely a result of too much exercise, in most cases.

Pain in a growing child can be a sign that he has a rheumatic infection, which could reach the heart if not treated quickly.

A child in such pain should be put to bed and the doctor called.

Hammer Toe. Deformity of bones of a toe, which causes it to bend into an inverted V shape. It occurs as a result of congenital defects such as club foot, or through badly fitting shoes.

The second toe is the usual one affected and because of pressure corns can develop. Surgery is needed to correct it.

Hangover. Unpleasant after-effects that can follow too much alcohol. As it is a poison which affects the entire system, the body takes time to recover from alcohol.

The hangover feeling may include upset stomach, dizziness, headache, thirst and feelings of depression and anxiety.

Treatment: Common-sense remedies such as aspirin and paracetamol for headaches. (Never take them with or immediately after drinking alcohol). To relieve thirst, drink plenty of fluids. Poached or boiled eggs, bread in hot milk, cereals and milk are the sort of bland foods to soothe the stomach.

Avoid a possible hangover in future by drinking milk *before* you take a drink. Or take your alcohol with a meal only. Or drink lots of water afterwards.

Hay Fever. Inflammation inside the nose due to an allergy — such as seasonal sensitivity to pollen (May to July); dust, certain plants and grasses; even some foods.

Symptoms: Similar to those of a common cold, except there is no rise in temperature. The nose and eyelids become swollen and irritated, there is sneezing and watery discharge from nose and eyes.

Treatment: A series of injections — of a standardised pollen vaccine — to immunise the sufferer, can be obtained from a doctor. Doses should start in about January, followed by weekly injections increasing in strength. These should continue for a few years until the sufferer is desensitised. Most of the drugs which relieve hay fever are antihistamines. A new drug, sodium cromoglycate, is effective in controlling the inflammation.

Hay fever sufferers should try to avoid substances which accelerate the allergy. For example, people who change from feather-filled pillows to synthetic-foam pillows usually find their symptoms disappear.

Herpes. Inflammation of the skin with a crop of small blisters. They remain as blisters for two or three days, then dry, form a scab, and disappear in about a week.

Two different types of virus are responsible, they are commonly known as cold sore and shingles. The same virus that causes shingles in adults gives children chickenpox. Shingles, the more troublesome of the two, is said to be caused by a virus which attacks the nerve roots.

Symptoms: A generally unwell feeling, a burning pain in the region of the affected nerve, most often on the abdomen. There may be a fever. At first the skin is red and sore then blisters appear round the affected part, which swells a little. After about five days the blisters begin to dry and a scab forms over them. There may be some residual pitting and scarring, though with careful treatment this can be avoided.

Certain forms of shingles may affect the eye nerves in the head, which means blisters may form on the face and sometimes the scalp. The eye may be inflamed and need careful nursing.

Treatment: Rest is essential. The first few days should be spent in bed. When an eruption appears it should be covered with a collodion dressing to prevent further infection and friction. Otherwise it should be kept dry by using talcum powder. If the pain is severe the doctor may give an injection. Analgesic tablets may be given if the pain is less troublesome, such as codeine, particularly if the sufferer is getting disturbed sleep.

A doctor should always be consulted in cases of shingles.

Hypertension. High blood pressure. When the heart pumps normally it works up a fluid pressure in the blood, sufficient to force it round the circulation system. In hypertension, this pressure is too high for the body's needs. The result is a strain of the heart, which has to pump harder to do its job. Gradually, small blood cells in the eyes and kidneys are affected, and this sets off a chain of events in which the vulnerable kidneys cause an increase in the blood pressure.

Hardening of the arteries (arteriosclerosis), kidney complaints, circulation disease, tumours of the adrenal glands, brain disease, may cause high blood pressure.

Strokes and thrombosis happen more often in people with high blood pressure.

Symptoms: These are slow to show. But shortness of breath, because of the strain on the heart, blurred vision, from damage to the back of the eyes, are signs that it needs urgent treatment.

Treatment: Doctors agree that lowering high blood pressure prolongs life. Sometimes the victim is overweight, and losing weight does reduce the blood pressure. Anti-hypersensitives, or drugs to reduce pressure, are often prescribed in addition to sedatives.

Rest is essential and it is also essential to give up smoking.

Hypochondria. Incessant worry about health or the possibility of something going wrong with the body. This abnormal fear gives rise to constant concern, and often depression, that there *is* something wrong. All the person's thoughts centre obsessively on it. The tiniest symptoms cause alarm and fear of some dread disease. When these are explained away, the hypochrondriac dreams up some other reasons to take its place.

This phobia is often coupled with other symptoms in someone extremely emotional or overwrought.

Hysterectomy. Removal of a woman's womb by surgery. Sometimes the entire womb is removed, but if medically possible the neck of the womb (cervix) is left in place. The ovaries and vagina are left in position in both operations, so that sexual desire and ability to make love are not diminished.

Where there is a serious disease, like cancer, the surgeon

performs a radical operation, and he does remove the ovaries, Fallopian Tubes and the upper part of the vagina. Some surgeons remove the ovaries in any woman who is past the menopause.

Most usual reason for a hysterectomy is the presence of fibroids (non-cancerous tumours) in the womb. These can cause heavy bleeding during a woman's periods — a sign that something is wrong inside. Quite often the womb becomes so large it interferes with the bladder and bowel functions. Excessive bleeding in itself during a woman's periods may prompt this operation, where a D and C (dilatation and curettage — widening the neck of the womb, scraping the womb lining) has failed. Again, pre-cancerous cells may be discovered during a cervical smear test — sparing the woman from developing actual cancer. But necessitating partial removal of the womb, depending on the extent of the diseased tissues.

Cancer of the neck of the womb is another reason for a hysterectomy, usually a radical one. Radiotherapy *may* be sufficient in dealing with this condition, again depending on how extensive the diseased area is.

Most women stay in hospital at least two weeks and can resume light housework in about two to three months. Heavy lifting and hard work should be left alone. In any case most women take about a year to really get back to their old selves.

Because not only is this a big operation (though no longer as feared as it used to be), it can disturb a woman's psyche and cause depression. Once she is fitter in herself, this despondency vanishes and she will feel less worried about the effects of her health, feminity, family and sexual activity.

In most cases, women experience a startling improvement in their general health, and have a new sparkle.

Hysteria. An unconscious action of the inner mind which induces the signs and symptoms usually seen in disease.

An hysterical person really does feel his symptoms are due to illness. But often it is a defence mechanism against a situation which is too hard to take. Hysteria can simulate a physical or mental disorder — for instance, deafness, blindness, dumbness, paralysis, fainting fits, and loss of memory.

It has been seen to break out when a group of teenage girls mob a pop star. This is an outbreak of heavy breathing, or panting, a sort of frenzy brought on by 'emotional fever'.

Hysterotomy. This is when a surgeon cuts into the womb, as in a Caesarian Section, to deliver a baby.

Impotence. A man who cannot achieve an erection, and so is unable to complete the sex act. Not to be confused with sterility, the condition when a man cannot produce sperm cells to become a father. The impotent man may produce perfectly healthy sperm cells, but cannot gain sexual satisfaction.

As a man grows older, his sex appetite tends to wane anyway, but that is *not* impotence.

There are many reasons for impotence. Most are emotional. A deep-rooted reason emanating from early life, such as a heavy-handed upbringing, a mother fixation, inability to assume a male role, even an adolescent rebuff from a girl that caused an in-built inferiority complex. Insecurity, depression, addiction to alcohol or drugs, job and money worries — all can impede a man emotionally and so inhibit him sexually.

Occasionally, the reason is physical. A man's sex organs may be deformed or be insufficient to have intercourse, or there may be a thyroid deficiency or a chronic disease like anaemia or diabetes.

Confidential advice can be obtained at one of many psycho-sexual clinics run by the Family Planning Association, 27 Mortimer Street, London W1.

Incontinence. Inability to retain urine or control the bowel movements. It is not unusual in older people, children, those who are very ill or recovering from a serious operation.

Incontinence can happen at any age, due perhaps to leakage through laughing, crying or coughing too much. Even excessive indulgence in sex can cause it.

A woman's pelvic muscles stretch in childbirth and in later years incontinence may be the result, during or after the menopause.

Treatment: Usually an operation to repair the strained muscles. Older people who don't have the operation should refrain from taking refreshments too near to bedtime. They may also get a course of drugs from the doctor.

Very young children don't have sufficient muscle control so often they cannot hold themselves. No child should be scolded for wetting himself, or soiling his nappy. Sympathy and good timing will win in the end.

Indigestion. A disturbance in the digestive system. But it is a term used lightly, just as people refer to stomach pain or upset tummy.

There *is* such a condition as indigestion, due perhaps to eating under emotional stress, over-eating, not eating enough, not chewing properly, swallowing food or drinks too quickly, heavy smoking. And there are foods which to some people are 'indigestible' — such as cucumber, cheese, fried or highly spiced dishes. Yet they eat them and suffer the discomforts of indigestion.

However, with its belching, feeling of fullness, nausea, cramp, constipation or diarrhoea, indigestion may well be a symptom of something much more serious. Persistent or recurring indigestion should not go unheeded. It is important to see a doctor.

Treatment: Simple indigestion can be avoided by not eating certain foods, and adopting sensible eating habits. The best way of getting rid of it is by taking a teaspoonful of baking soda in water — it will relieve the feeling and the discomfort by breaking wind. An anti-acid medicine, such as aluminium hydroxide or magnesium trisilicate can be soothing.

Infertility. Inability of a couple to have children. The fault may lie in the man or the woman. Only tests by a gynaecologist or at special fertility clinics will identify which partner is infertile.

When a woman is unable to conceive there may be a weakness or infection in the Fallopian Tubes, or they may simply be blocked. Infection of the lining of the womb is also possible. Both these parts of the reproductive organs must be healthy for conception to occur. The trouble may be a disorder of the hormone-producing endocrine glands. Or, as often happens, it may be purely emotional.

In a man, examination will prove whether his semen contains normal sperm cells or enough of them. He may be impotent, and because he cannot complete the sex act, conception fails to take place.

Some couples in this situation who desperately want children can try artificial insemination.

The woman can either have her husband's healthy sperm (if he is fertile but impotent) deposited by syringe into her vagina, when she is at her most fertile.

Or, when the husband's sperm is weaker or produced in smaller amounts than normal, it can be preserved over a period of time in a frozen state. When there is sufficient it can be inserted into the woman in the same way.

Or, if the husband is sterile, the donor can be another man. This is what is known as A.I.D. In this situation the doctor clears the donor (who remains anonymous) as far as health, sound hereditary and blood compatibility are concerned.

Influenza. Acute infectious disease caused by a virus. One virus is never quite the same as the previous one, and many different strains have been identified.

Often the name of the place where a particular epidemic starts gives its name to the strain — as in 1957, when severe Asian flu swept across Europe. Hong Kong flu, a relatively mild version, was first pinpointed in Hong Kong in 1968. It spread to Europe during the following months.

As it is certainly infectious and has an incubation period of only one to four days, flu spreads rapidly. The virus enters the body in drops of air and it is transmitted partly by coughing and sneezing.

Symptoms: They vary. But usually there is a headache behind the eyes, loss of appetite, chill, catarrh, fever, weakness, shivering, general aches and pains, inflammation of the nose and throat. In the nervous form, there may be delirium, sleeplessness and extreme exhaustion.

There are several versions of the disease:

1. Epidemic form, now thought of as the true influenza virus.

2. Respiratory form, which may lead to bronchitis, pleurisy and pneumonia.

3. Gastro-intestinal type, commonly referred to as 'gastric flu'.

4. Nervous form, which may occur as the main complaint, or as a result of the first three types.

Influenza weakens the body's defences against germs,

which is why old people and those with heart disease or chest problems can be hard hit.

Treatment: Send for the doctor right away. Even with the slightest symptoms a patient should stay in bed to avoid spreading the infection.

Rest in bed is vital if the illness takes the epidemic form, if only to prevent danger to the heart. The bedroom should be warm, fully ventilated, but free from draughts. The patient should stay in bed three to four days or, unless there are other complications, until the temperature is back to normal. It is foolish to fight on bravely and continue normal activities, because of the risk of complications setting in.

Solid food should be avoided, but the patient should take lots of warm drinks. Early on in simple cases, take an aspirin with Dover's powder and a glass of water, night and morning, for 24 to 48 hours. This should be followed by a hot drink of rum or whisky and milk, or whisky, hot lemon and demerara sugar. These remedies encourage perspiration, relieve headache and limb pains, and induce a restful sleep.

There is a vaccine that can be injected to give temporary immunity against flu. But this is useless once symptoms have developed.

Ingrowing Toe-nail. This is when the nail of the big toe, usually, tends to curve into the flesh on the sides of the toe, instead of growing straight out. It is generally caused by badly fitting, narrow shoes and neglect in cutting the toe-nails. Untreated, this can be very painful, with inflammation, soreness and possible discharge.

Treatment: A doctor or preferably a chiropodist should be consulted. The overgrowth of skin will be diminished, the nail cut evenly and medicated gauze plugs used to press back the overhanging skin. The groove is then dusted with antiseptic powder.

Quite often, in simple cases, the chiropodist will file the surface of the toe-nail, which has probably grown quite thick, to make it flatter and more flexible. This prevents the edges being forced into the flesh.

If these methods are impossible, then in rare cases surgical removal of the nail is the only successful treatment.

Jaundice. Not a disease in itself but a symptom of some other disorder. Most noticeable feature is that the sufferer develops a yellow skin and the whites of the eyes also become yellow. This discolouration is because the blood contains too much of a certain constituent of bile. These are the three main reasons for jaundice:

1. Liver disease, whereby the liver cells are unable to deal with the bile in the normal way. Cirrhosis, infectious hepatitis, serum hepatitis, and Weil's disease can all cause jaundice.

2. Blockage of the bile duct. This often happens because a gallstone has formed in the gall bladder and passed into the bile duct where it causes pain and inflammation, or jaundice. An operation may be necessary to remove a stone if it becomes affected.

3. Excessive breakdown of red blood cells (haemolytic anaemia), which can happen in a newborn baby, particularly the child of a Rhesus-Positive father and Rh-Negative mother, or in someone who has had a transfusion of the wrong blood type.

A doctor must be consulted right away to establish and treat the basic disorder.

Laparoscopy. Technique of making a tiny insertion into the abdomen, near the navel, and inserting an optical instrument called a laparoscope. Many surgeons now use this method of viewing the ovaries and Fallopian Tubes and also when performing a sterilisation operation in a woman.

Laryngitis. Inflammation of the voice-box (larynx). The acute condition can follow a cold or flu. Or it may be due to over-use of the voice in actors, singers or preachers. Occasionally it occurs in diptheria.

Symptoms: Usually it is accompanied by a dry cough, hoarseness, a tickle in the throat, pain in swallowing. Eventually the voice may disappear entirely.

Treatment: The patient must stay in a warm, well centilated room, with no draughts. The atmosphere must not be too dry. Warm, soothing drinks, occasionally sucking ice, will help relieve pain. If there is difficulty in swallowing, custards, milk puddings, junkets may be infinitely easier than liquids.

Aspirin and Dover's powders will relieve pain and congestion. Kaolin poultices or ice packs will soothe externally. Inhaling Friar's Balsam frequently (one teaspoonful to a pint of boiling water) relieves the larynx. The patient should stay indoors after inhaling, because of an increased risk of a chill or bronchitis.

If the condition doesn't disappear in a couple of days, send for the doctor who will prescribe a soothing linctus and may possibly order a throat spray with penicillin in normal saline solution.

Laxative. Medicine to help empty the bowels. There are several types:

1. Bulk laxatives, which increase the solid matter in the motions. As the Western diet is so refined, with white bread, white sugar, etc., it contains precious little indigestible waste matter. Many doctors believe 'roughage', such as green vegetables, brown bread, cereals, should be eaten to keep bowel movements healthy.

2. Drugs. These force the intestinal muscles to contract, forcing waste matter along the lower intestines. Senna pods, steeped in water, or tablets containing senna are the most widely used.

3. Osmotic laxatives. These increase the stools by causing the intestines to retain some of the water normally absorbed into the blood. Epsom salts (magnesium sulphate) and Glauber's salts (sodium sulphate) are the most used.

Never take a laxative regularly for constipation, which can usually be overcome by a good diet and healthy living. Never take a laxative when there is pain in the abdomen. This may be a symptom of something seriously wrong, and the laxative might rupture for instance the inflamed part of the intestine.

Mastectomy. Surgical removal of the breast, most often to treat breast cancer.

Treatment is usually a success, *providing* a woman doesn't delay seeing her doctor and/or a specialist as soon as she finds a lump in her breast (See Breast, Inspection of).

There are various means of detecting whether a lump is malignant, by:

1. *Palpation* (hand examination).

2. *Thermography* (the patient sits in front of a photoscanning machine, which shows the inside of her breasts

like a relief map, and the extra-sensitive camera identifies any abnormalities).

3. *Mammography* (low dose X-ray).

The surgeon, after an initial biopsy (removal of part of the tumour tissue and examination under a microscope to determine whether the growth is malignant or not) will decide what form the mastectomy operation takes. This will depend on his own opinion, and the type and extent of the cancer:

1. *Partial* mastectomy, removing only that part of the tissue which is diseased.

2. *Total* mastectomy, removal of the entire breast.

3. *Radical* mastectomy, removal of the breast, the muscle underneath and the tissue in the armpit.

Afterwards X-ray treatment is given to eliminate any further cancerous tissue. Whatever form of operation is performed, the patient has a good outlook, particularly if she has sought early treatment.

Artificial breasts of various forms, and adaptable to match perfectly, are available. A woman will be asked to go for a regular check-up at the hospital where she had her operation. Psychologically, it may take her a little more time to recover than from the physical effects.

Counselling, both on the physical and psychological aspects of mastectomy, can be obtained from Mrs Betty Westgate, herself once a mastectomy patient, founder of The Mastectomy Association, 1 Colworth Road, Croydon, Surrey, CRO 7AD.

Mastitis. Inflammation of the breast, with a feeling of pain and sensitivity. The usual cause is a hormone imbalance or an infection. Sometimes a mother experiences it while nursing her newborn baby. This may be the result of poor breast hygiene, infection, or an abscess.

The mother usually has to stop breast-feeding her baby. Antibiotics soon clear up this condition.

Masturbation. Once considered dangerous to the mind and body, masturbation is simply manipulation of the genitals to get an orgasm.

It is sometimes used by nervous people as a sexual outlet to relieve tension, or in the absence of a partner. But it shows an extreme state of nervous disorder if done to excess and may indicate a need for psychological counselling.

Measles. Generally a contagious disease of childhood, which shows itself in a pink rash on the face, neck and body. Catching it in childhood usually means immunity for life, which is why it is so rare in adults.

Symptoms: Sneezing, coughing, running nose, sore eyes, a fever in which the temperature may reach 106 degrees F. The rash comprising many small red spots appears from three to five days after the other symptoms show themselves, and lasts from four to seven days. The fever normally drops when the rash appears. Complete recovery takes two to four weeks.

Treatment: Send for the doctor, who will soon diagnose mealses from small white-centred red spots in the mouth and inside the cheeks.

Isolate the patient in a well ventilated room. His eyes may be sensitive to light, so draw the curtains. Keep him on a light diet during the fever. The patient should stay in bed until his temperature returns to normal and he can then get up. But he must be careful, as anyone with measles is very susceptible to colds, or even pneumonia.

Since 1968, with the introduction of a measles vaccine in Britain, the disease has declined dramatically. Deaths have dropped by almost two-thirds.

Babies should be vaccinated against measles when they are about nine months old. A single injection produces immunity for life. The baby or child may develop mild measles symptoms 10 days after being vaccinated. Don't worry, but call the doctor.

Migraine. Recurring, usually severe headache, sometimes accompanied by loss of appetite, nausea and vomiting. This disorder sometimes runs in families. Most often it attacks one side of the head and can affect speech and make the sufferer feel weak while it lasts.

Classic migraine may involve loss of speech, a change of mood, and vision so disturbed the sufferer is blinded by flashing or patterned lights. This causes great discomfort and momentary panic.

Common migraine is usually no more than a headache, with nausea and vomiting.

Some women get it in the week before their periods. It

may be brought on by alcohol or eating certain foods. Scientists have discovered that it may be due to a chemical upset in the body's nervous system.

Drugs are used to combat migraine and to prevent it: simple analgesics like aspirin and paracetamol or ones specially for migraine, such as ergotamine tartrate or anti-emetic drugs.

Sufferers can get information and advice from The Migrain Trust, 23 Queen Square, London WC1 N 3AY.

Miscarriage. Accidental loss of the foetus from the womb before the seventh month of pregnancy. After that time, the baby can survive outside the womb. If expelled in the last two months of pregnancy, this is *premature labour.*

A miscarriage should not be confused with an *abortion,* which is a deliberate expulsion of the foetus from the womb.

In most cases, a miscarriage is the body's way of rejecting a foetus which is damaged or defective in some way. And had it reached maturity the baby would have been abnormal. But the exact reason cannot be explained in half of all miscarriages.

In some cases the foetus has incorrectly planted itself in the Fallopian tube instead of in the womb and when it gets too big (after 8 to 12 weeks) may rupture the tube, again causing a miscarriage. Kidney trouble, veneral disease, a disorder of the endocrine glands, may also be responsible for a miscarriage.

Symptoms: Bleeding from the vagina is the signal. All cases of bleeding should be reported right away to the doctor. If the bleeding continues and is heavy and accompanied by rhythmic waves of cramp, then a miscarriage is pretty definite.

Morning Sickness. During the early months of pregnancy, usually the first two to three, a woman will experience nausea and vomiting when she gets up. If it is very bad it is called emesis and can be treated with drugs. Some lucky pregnant women don't get morning sickness at all.

Multiple Sclerosis. A disease, cause unknown, which attacks the nerve linings in various parts of the brain and spinal cord. The nerve tissues are damaged and replaced by scar tissue, so those nerves stop working. The sufferer is usually a young adult.

Symptoms: Impaired or double vision; weakness, pins and needles, difficulty in walking. The symptoms come and go, lasting a few days or several months. Gradually the victim becomes disabled.

Skilled medical treatment can help patients lead a fairly normal life.

Information and help can be obtained from The Multiple Sclerosis Society, 4 Tachbrook Street, London SW1 V1SJ.

Mumps. Infectious disease, caused by a virus, in which the parotid glands, situated below the ears, become enlarged and inflamed. It occurs mostly in children.

Symptoms: Two or three weeks after infection the patient complains of feeling ill, or the first sign may be pain and difficulty in eating; the tonsils and throat may also be inflamed. Sometimes only the glands on one side of the face swell up initially and it may be another two days before the other side becomes affected. The complaint lasts from four to six days. After about eight days from the first symptom the patient is all right again.

Treatment: The disease does not call for much treatment except rest in bed. Diet should be soft enough to avoid painful mastication: egg, fish and milk dishes are suitable but the patient is not allowed condiments or highly seasoned food.

Affected persons rarely contract the disease a second time.

As it occasionally happens that glands other than the parotid glands are affected, particularly the testicles in males, and more rarely the ovaries in females, and sometimes the pancreas, the doctor should always be called when the disease first becomes apparent.

Neuralgia. Normally a severe inflammation and pain in the nerves of the face, lower back and legs. In the face it can momentarily irritate the forehead, cheek, lips, jaw and tongue and cause great pain.

Sometimes it is because false teeth do not fit properly, or the natural teeth don't meet comfortably. An attack may be triggered off by eating, speaking or brushing the teeth.

A doctor will prescribe drugs to relieve the pain.

Neuritis. Exposure to cold or wet, injury, or a particular job may cause this nerve inflammation. In its most severe form, where several nerves are affected, it can be set off by alcohol, diabetes, severe flu, chronic arsenic or lead poisoning, malnutrition. Occasionally there is some degree of paralysis.

Symptoms: Tingling or numbness, loss of ability in the lower arms and legs, especially in the later stages, and severe shooting pains along the course of the nerves, which may give rise to agonising pains. The skin becomes smooth and glossy, and the nails brittle and cracked in chronic cases.

Treatment: Rest in bed is vital. The doctor should be called and the cause of the trouble removed. Large doses of Vitamin B1 by mouth and by injection may shorten an attack and speed up recovery.

Chronic alcoholism and diabetes, and the neuritis caused by metallic poisons will need the doctor's immediate attention and advice.

Obesity. Excessive accumulation of fat in various parts of the body. It can occur in childhood, but more frequently in middle age.

Usual cause is over-eating, especially of fatty foods and carbohydrates, and heavy beer drinking. Lack of exercise is a minor factor. Occasionally obesity is due to a glandular disorder. Because of it, the heart and circulation system have to work much harder. The fat person becomes more liable to get arthritis, backache, flat feet, diabetes and hardening of the arteries.

Piles *(Haemorrhoids).* Enlarged or varicose veins of the lower part of the back passage. When they become inflamed and swollen they cause great pain, and there is often bleeding.

There is no obvious cause, but some result from pressure on the anal area, caused by straining to relieve constipation, or too many laxatives used too often. Piles can develop during pregnancy, when the foetus pushes against the abdominal wall. A tumour or large cyst may also cause pressure and piles.

Ordinary piles can be extremely painful when they become strangulated or thrombosis occurs.

Treatment: First, treat the cause of the complaint. If it is constipation, take liquid paraffin. A short-term measure to relieve pain is to apply cold water on a tissue or cloth to the anal area. A warm bath several times a day helps relax the spasm that sometimes develops in the muscles and the back passage.

After washing, apply a soothing ointment of zinc and camphor or an astringent with witch hazel ointment. A soothing and astringent suppository at night is of great benefit.

A doctor may recommend the injection of a special fluid around the large veins to shrivel them up.

External piles should be treated by injection or operated on by a doctor or surgeon, who should be consulted as soon as the condition appears.

Rheumatism. Disorders of various kinds involving pain in the joints and bones, and the tissues supporting them.

Rheumatism may be the result of theumatoid arthritis, gout, osteo-arthritis. Of these, rheumatic fever is due to a specific germ which can damage the heart as well as the joints of young adults, and often follows an earlier infection such as impetigo, or tonsilitis. Gout is caused by faulty metabolism. (See under Gout).

Rubella *(German Measles).* Three-day measles characterised by a contagious pink rash on the face, neck and body. It occurs in epidemics and may disappear for years. One attack usually gives life-long immunity.

German measles has become notorious in the cases of expectant mothers. If in the first three months of pregnancy a woman contracts rubella, the chances are quite high that the baby will have serious defects at birth. Occasionally the foetus dies. Induced abortion may be recommended as an alternative. If the woman becomes pregnant again, the new baby will not be threatened by the mother's previous infection.

An effective vaccine against German measles is available. It should be given to a girl when she is about 13.

Symptoms: These are mild. The victim may be unaware he has an illness until a rash appears, two to three weeks after exposure to the infection. There may be a fever and tenderness under the armpit, in the neck and groin. Recovery is natural. No specific treatment is needed.

Scarlet Fever. An infectious disease which may attack individuals of all ages, but is generally confined to children between 2 and 15 years.

Symptoms: First signs are usually headache and vomiting, frequently accompanied by sore .throat, diarrhoea and a high temperature. The skin is dry, the tongue furred and the face is generally flushed. A rash of small bright red dots, close together, appears after 24 hours, beginning on the sides of the neck and chest and spreading quickly all over the body, except round the mouth, which is usually pale.

Treatment: Isolate and send immediately for the doctor.

In straightforward cases Scarlet Fever ceases to be infectious after about 3 weeks, and this may be confirmed by the absence of the causative streptoccocci from the culture of throat swabs. Since the availability of the sulphonamides and penicillin, complications have become rare.

An attack of Scarlet Fever confers permanent immunity.

Sciatica. A very common form of neuritis which attacks with excruciating pain the sciatic nerve — the major nerve which passes from the lower back into the legs. The middle aged and old are the usual victims.

There are various conditions which may bring it on: strain of the lower back; exposure to cold or wet; injury and chronic arthritis, in the lower spine area; a slipped disc in the spine pressing on the sciatic nerve. Gout and rheumatism can be responsible. Chronic alcoholics may also develop sciatica. In women backward displacement of the womb may cause it.

Symptoms: Pain passing from the lower back into the back of the thigh and often down to the ankles. Stretching and exercise make it worse, and sleep is difficult. The area is tender when touched and often obstinate to treatment. In chronic cases, there may be wasting of the thigh and bottom muscles.

Treatment: Rest in bed. The legs should be kept still and heat applied to the area in pain. A doctor should be called, and he will prescribe sedatives and possibly advise physiotherapy and certain exercises.

Sickness *(Air, Train, Sea, etc.).* Most seasoned travellers know how their system reacts and will have found a remedy for themselves by trial and error.

Nausea and vomiting are the most usual problem experienced by some people when they travel in a boat, plane, train or even in a bus or car. Some get sick in a swing or a lift. The rhythmical movement of a boat may cause it and if there is no fresh air, or unpleasant fumes, as in a car with closed windows, then the reaction is worsened.

The cause stems from the ear, where the balancing mechanism is upset and the result is travel sickness. Here are some tips for the touchy traveller:

Treatment: The day before the journey take a laxative and glucose. An hour or two before the actual trip, have a light meal with strong coffee and plenty of glucose. Barley sugar, glucose or chewing gum may help in air travel. On sea trips, if possible, get a position near the middle of the boat away from the sides.

Lie on a chair covered with a rug or flat on the back, and sleep or close the eyes. A band or belt evenly tied round the upper abdomen is also a good preventative measure.

When vomiting or nausea persist, brandy and hot black coffee or weak China tea give relief. Iced champagne, if available, sips of soda water with a slice of lemon, or brandy and soda may relieve the sickness.

There are many anti-sickness tablets available, some containing anti-histamines. But *do* read the instructions carefully. Such tablets are not advisable if a woman is pregnant. If she is on the birth pill, the constituents of certain anti-sickness tablets may cancel the effectiveness of The Pill.

Tonsilitis. Acute sore throat and inflammation of the tonsils (a pair of oval tissues which protect the throat from invading germs), due to infection by various germs. Sometimes the tonsils become a chronic focus of repeated infection and a doctor may advise that they are removed surgically. This is often done simultaneously with infected adenoids.

Symptoms: Sore throat, pain and difficulty in swallowing, shivering, possibly pains in the back, a rise in temperature, furred tongue, bad breath, constipation, tonsils red and swollen, pain in the glands of the neck. The illness may last up to a week.

The tonsils may become so infected that they discharge pus, ulcerate or produce an abscess (quinsey). There may be inflammation of the middle ear and even acute rheumatism.

Treatment: Call a doctor, and stay in bed. Hot poultices or kaolin poultices can be applied to the neck. Use antiseptic mouth wash and gargle as often as possible. Antibiotics will prevent quinsey, avoid other complications, and aid recovery. The doctor may take a swab to rule out the presence of diphtheria, (now a rare disease in this country).

Tranquilliser. Drug taken in the prescribed dose, which quietens an anxious or agitated mind, and which doesn't cause drowsiness or interfere with a person's normal responses.

Since they were introduced in the 1950's, these drugs have helped a lot in severe emotional stress and mental disorders. Tranquillisers mean a person can lead a relatively normal life when without them he would be unable to function.

One of the original tranquillisers, Rauwolfia, was derived from a well known Indian snake-root plant. As well as its use in treating mental illness, it can lower the blood pressure and relieve withdrawal symptoms in drug addicts. Today, however, most tranquillisers are synthetic — best known are, Equanil (a meprobamate), Librium (a chlordiazepoxide) and Valium (a diazepam), which are fairly mild.

Tranquillisers may calm the mind, but they do not *cure* the real underlying cause of the anxiety. There are some side-effects, and they can be habit-forming. Tranquillisers should always be taken under close medical supervision.

Tuberculosis. With the advent of drug treatment, tuberculosis is no longer the big killer disease it was 20 years ago.

Tuberculosis is an infectious disease which comes in two forms. One affects the lungs. The other affects the voice box, the bones, joints, glands, intestines, kidneys and nervous system.

The disease is usually contracted by breathing in germs or eating contaminated food or liquids. Once upon a time, before eradication of TB in cattle and widespread pasteurisation of milk, the disease could be carried from infected cows.

People living in overcrowded cities can still be exposed to tuberculosis germs, which are able to survive in phlegm which has dried after being coughed up, and in dust, for some time. But the infection, being mild, gives them an immunity against the disease. The circumstances in which

TB germs gain a foothold is where people are under-nourished and living in overcrowded, insanitary conditions which weaken the body's natural defences.

Early signs and symptoms:

1. No cold or cough, especially if accompanied by phlegm, should be ignored. If there is a general feeling of apathy or a person is 'run down', seek medical advice and ask the doctor if he advises an X-ray.

2. Never waste the opportunity of a chest X-ray if it occurs in the place where you work or live.

3. Report any of these signs to your doctor immedi-ately — loss of weight, night sweating, rise in temperature and pulse rate, which is higher in the evening than in the morning, a tired feeling or tendency to tire easily after exertion, digestive disturbances, any sign of blood when you cough up phlegm.

Treatment: Many patients can be treated at home, although a cure may be started in hospital in certain cases. The three chief drugs used to combat TB are streptomycin, isoniazid (INH) and para-aminosalicylic acid (PAS). So effective is treatment today that many of the old sanatoriums and special hospitals are now used for other purposes through lack of patients.

General Prevention: Make sure your diet is balanced and that you eat sufficient food containing the necessary vita-mins, especially A and D. No slimming diet should ever be embarked on without first consulting your doctor. Fresh air, particularly in the bedroom, cleanliness in the home as well as reasonable living space, outdoor exercise, the use of only pasturised milk, are essential.

Mass X-ray units touring the country, X-raying the chest of all who are willing, have done much to uncover early cases, which are so easily cured. Routine testing of school-children with BCG vaccine, and the great advance made in treatment with such drugs as streptomycin and PAS, have transformed the whole picture.

Varicose Veins. These arise through a deficiency of the valves of the veins, a weakness of the walls of the blood vessels. The condition is aggravated by long periods of standing, hard training, or severe exertion. Women, older people and those who are overwieght tend to get them more often than others. There is a tendency for varicose veins to recur in families.

Pressure outside the veins also contributes, such as tight girdles, constant constipation, and some tumours of the pelvis.

Varicose veins often first appear in women during pregnancy. If they are already present, they may become considerably worse. The veins need particular attention in pregnancy as there is a risk of inflammation, or phlebitis.

Symptoms: The veins become abnormally wide, knotted and elongated. They look blue under the skin and are unsightly. The limbs feel heavy and the ankles puffy. There is itchiness and skin inflammation, and the feet may become cold and numb.

Complications can arise, such as phlebitis, thrombosis, varicose eczema, varicose ulcer and haemorrhage from a burst or ulcerated vein.

Treatment: In mild cases, a painless injection is made into the affected veins, which eventually close and have their functions taken over by other blood vessels. Sometimes injections are very successful, but in other cases they have little effect.

Most effective treatment, in severe cases, is surgery. The lining of the major affected vein is removed. Weak veins that connect with it are tied off by a process known as ligation. After the operation the blood makes its way to the heart through other veins.

Lots of rest, with the legs slightly raised, can help control slight cases. Elastic stockings help prevent swelling, and walking helps by stimulating the circulation in the legs.

Venereal Disease. Various disorders of the genitals in men and women and transmitted through sexual contact. They include, *syphilis* (the most serious), *chancroid* or *soft core*, and *gonorrhoea* (the most common). Less troublesome but still infectious are, *vaginal trichomonas* (in a woman) and *non-specific urethritis* (in a man).

Venereal diseases, particularly gonorrhoea, are vastly on the increase in Britain, where one in about 200 people needs treatment. Although new drugs can cure most types, if the diseases are discovered quickly, VD is still very dangerous because it is a *hidden* disease.

Gonorrhoea: the most common, is more serious than people realise. In a man it causes a painful, burning sensation on passing urine, and there may be a discharge of yellowish pus from the penis.

In a woman, there are usually no early symptoms. Any pus or germs mingle in ordinary female secretions and pass out of the body unnoticed. There *may* be inflammation of the passage from the bladder and pain when passing water. Later there will be abdominal pain and fever, due to inflammation of the Fallopian Tubes. If a woman doesn't get treatment these tubes may become permanently blocked and she may be unable to have a baby. If she does have a child while she has gonorrhoea the baby may be blind.

Syphilis: Untreated, this is *very* serious, and can affect men and women in the same way.

First sign is a painless sore or ulcer, which usually appears in or near the sex organs three to six weeks after the infection has occurred. The ulcer is full of syphilis germs which can infect any minute crack in the skin of anyone coming into contact.

In a man the ulcer is easily seen, but in a woman it may be hidden inside the vagina so that she knows nothing about it. After days or weeks the ulcers in both cases disappear. But some weeks later there is a generalised illness, with fever, sore throat, headache and a rash (this is secondary syphilis). These also go away.

The germs may be unnoticed. But if untreated, they stay very active and by now will have reached the brain, nervous system, eyes, liver and heart. They can weaken, damage or cripple almost every organ and may eventually cause paralysis, blindness, insanity and death. This is the third stage of the disease.

A woman with untreated syphilis who becomes pregnant can pass the germ into the blood stream of her baby, so that it is born dead or diseased.

There are several other diseases which may be spread by indiscriminate sex. Most common and important is *non-specific urethritis* (or NSU). It produces a discharge in a man, but women are usually carriers of the germ and have no symptoms.

This infection can lead to diseases of the joints, eye disease and inflammation of the sex organs. Some of the other conditions produce discharge in women. One of the commonest being *Trichomonas*. The man may be the carrier and not know that he is infected.

Another disease, thrush *(Candidiasis)* usually produces itching and soreness in women.

Anyone who has recently had sexual contact with a new partner and is suspicious that he or she may have contracted a disease, can obtain treatment — very discreetly — at any of about 250 special clinics in Britain. Many are attached to hospitals.

Precautions: Couples who are faithful to each other have nothing to worry about. But if you sleep with someone you don't know, or change partners, you are taking a chance — and taking a chance of passing VD to someone you love as well as getting it yourself.

The risks are not so great if the man wears a sheath (French letter). But he must be careful not to touch the woman's sex organs before he puts the sheath on, and must handle it as little as possible afterwards. Washing the genitals with soap and water after intercourse also reduces risk. But none of these precautions is 100 per cent certain.

The best way to avoid getting VD is to be sure the person you are having sex with is not affected.

Wart *(Verruca).* Small hard benign (non-cancerous) growths on and rooted to the skin, and caused by a virus. They can often be found on the fingers, hands, elbows and face.

Hard warts: Occur mainly on the sole of the foot at the base of the toes. Because of pressure from standing and walking hard skin builds up. Highly infectious, they are often picked up in gymnasiums and swimming baths, which is why they are most common in children.

Soft warts: These occur on the genitals and around the anus, causing itching and discomfort. Some are cauliflower shaped and others are attached to the skin by a thin stalk.

Treatment: Several methods can remove a wart. A doctor may cauterise with an electric needle or chemicals, or freeze it with dry ice (solid carbon dioxide). This is how a chiropodist will deal with a foot verruca. Sometimes minor surgery is necessary, including X-ray, or an injection of smallpox vaccine.

Never try to remove a wart yourself. If a wart changes shape or several suddenly appear, then this could indicate a disorder. See a doctor.

OUTLINES OF FIRST AID

Because of the increasing number and serious nature of accidents of all kinds, the responsibility of the first aider is greater today than ever.

First Aid is treatment given to a casualty:
- *to sustain life.*
- *to prevent the condition from getting worse.*
- *to help recovery.*

When dealing with any casualty first make a diagnosis. That is, find out what the injuries are, remembering that there may be several things wrong. It is no use treating a broken leg if the injured person is choking to death; nor bandaging a cut head if the casualty is bleeding to death from a deep wound in the thigh.

All the injuries must be assessed; the most dangerous treated first.

As you take charge, be calm and give the conscious casualty confidence by talking to him, listening to him and reassuring him. Check the safety of the casualties and yourself; check breathing and for bleeding and whether he or she is conscious. Get others to help. Tell them what they should do. If necessary, send for ambulance, police, fire brigade, or other help.

Now, how do you make a diagnosis?

This is done by getting the *history* of the accident either from the casualty or from witnesses; if the casualty is conscious you ask what is troubling him, and if he is unconscious you make an examination. In this way you will discover the *symptoms*. Then you look for signs of injury and *level of consciousness*.

So you base your diagnosis on these four things, the *history* of the casualty, the *symptoms*, the signs and the *level of consciousness*.

History. You learn a certain amount from using your eyes and ears and nose. You can *see* the smashed-up car or broken bicycle ... but listen carefully, for the casualty may say, 'I don't remember anything' or 'I hit the pavement and fell off'. But the witness may say, 'I saw the man slump over the steering wheel' or 'I saw the man fall off his bike and his head strike the pavement'. You can *smell* escaping gas, and so on. Don't forget, if there is a question of poisoning, to take care of any bottles of medicine or tablets you find at the scene of the accident. Both the doctor and the police will need to see them. And if the casualty is conscious, don't forget to look through the pockets or a handbag. There may be evidence that the casualty suffers from diabetes or other disease or is taking special drugs. For instance, a man or woman with a heart complaint usually carries treatment for just such an emergency.

Symptoms. These are what the casualty complains of — 'I feel cold'. 'I am in pain'. 'My arm is numb'. It can be faintness, nausea, thirst ... nobody knows better than the injured person exactly where, and how ill he feels. After all, it is *his* body that is in trouble.

Signs. The signs are what you find that varies from normal and means the casualty's condition is abnormal. The broken leg which is mis-shapen, the pallid face, the rapid pulse, the blue face, lips and inner sides of the eyelids, and nail beds of fingers and toes. All these are tell tale signs.

Level of consciousness. Any change of level is important. *Full consciousness* means the casualty can speak and answer questions normally. *Drowsiness* means he is easily roused, but lapses into an unconscious state. *Stupor*, can be roused with difficulty. The casualty will be aware of painful stimuli, such as a pin prick, but not answer when spoken to. *Coma*, cannot be roused by any stimuli.

Certain initial action can be taken. If the cause of the condition is still apparent, remove it — a log of wood on the casualty's thigh, contaminated clothing. *Or* remove the casualty from the cause — from fire, water, poisonous fumes, etc.

The Golden Rules of First Aid

1. Act quickly, quietly, methodically, and don't panic. Give priority to the most urgent conditions.

2. If breathing has stopped or is failing, clear the air passages and, if necessary, start emergency resuscitation.

3. Control bleeding.

4. Determine the level of consciousness.

5. Consider the possibility of poisoning.

6. Guard against shock. Remember that rapid removal to hospital is vital.

7. Reassure the casualty as necessary and those around him, to help lessen the anxiety. Handle the casualty gently at all times.

8. Position the casualty correctly.

9. Before moving the casualty, immobilise fractures and large wounds.

10. Don't take off any more clothing than is necessary. But don't hesitate to remove clothes to make a proper examination or to get at a wound.

11. Arrange immediately for the careful conveyance of the casualty, if necessary, to the care of his doctor or to a hospital. Watch and note any changes in his condition in the meantime.

Do *not* attempt too much.

Do *not* allow people to crowd round. This only hinders first aid and may make the casualty anxious or embarrassed.

Do *not* give anything by mouth to a casualty who is unconscious, who has a suspected internal injury, or who may shortly need an anaesthetic.

ACTION AT AN EMERGENCY

First, you must consider placing an unconscious casualty in the *recovery position* (once known as the coma position, and, earlier, as the three-quarters prone position); temporarily *control any continuous bleeding*, with the help of the casualty or others, if available; *restore breathing*, if necessary.

When sending for help make sure witnesses understand the message to be sent. Write it down if possible but certainly always get them to repeat it to you before actually sending it.

Priorities. Reduce to a minimum any danger to the casualty or yourself. In the case of — *electrocution:* switch off the current, and take precautions against electric shock — *fire:* move the casualty to safety — *gas and poisonous fumes:* turn off at source and remove casualty to fresh air. The urgent needs of the casualty will be his breathing: check that the air passage is clear, and that he is breathing. If not, start artificial respiration. Next his unconsciousness: place him in the recovery position, and check for serious bleeding and control it; raise the part if possible and if no fracture is suspected. Then, using all your senses to the maximum, look, speak, listen, feel and smell as you make your diagnosis. Let us first study the:

Conscious casualty
1. Look and weigh up the problem as you approach.
2. Ask him if he has pain and where it is. Examine that part first.
3. Ask him if he thinks there is anything else wrong.
4. Handle injured parts firmly but gently.
5. Make sure there are no injuries which may be masked by pain, by checking for tenderness and bleeding.
6. Examine the casualty carefully in a regular and methodical manner by running your hands gently but firmly over all parts of the body. Begin at the head and neck, then check the spine and trunk; the upper limbs and lower limbs. Always compare the abnormal parts with the normal side.
Then check: the colour of the skin, the nail beds and the inside of the eye-lids; the nature of the breathing, listen to it, is it fast, slow, irregular; smell the breath; count the pulse, noting its strength and rhythm; the temperature of the body, whether hot or cold to the touch.

Unconscious casualty
1. This is much more difficult and a thorough detailed examination is necessary.
2. Decide if he is breathing; if not, immediately start artificial respiration.
3. Examine over and under the casualty for dampness which might indicate bleeding. Stop any serious bleeding before going any further with the investigation.
4. Bear in mind the possibility of internal bleeding.
5. Establish the cause of unconsciousness by examining the breathing (rate and depth), pulse (rate and character),

face and skin (colour, temperature and condition), pupils of the eyes, head for injury, ears, eyes, nose and mouth for blood or other signs of injury.

This is how to turn an unconscious casualty into the recovery position.

1. Kneel by him and place both his arms close to his body.

2. Turn the casualty gently on his side (this may be easily done by grasping his clothes at the hip).

3. Draw up the upper arm until it makes a right angle with the body and bend the elbow.

4. Draw up the upper leg until the thigh makes a right angle with the body and bend the knee.

5. Draw out the underneath arm gently backwards to extend slightly behind his back.

6. Bend the undermost knee slightly.

By placing the limbs like this it provides the necessary stability to keep the casualty comfortable in the *recovery position*. With his head turned to one side the possibility of vomit causing drowning is eliminated.

BANDAGES AND DRESSINGS

A dressing is a protective covering applied to a wound to prevent infection, absorb discharge, control bleeding, avoid further injury.

The dressing should be sterile, that is germ free, if possible, and act as a filter restricting the entry of germs, which could infect the wound. A dressing may be a piece of sterile surgical gauze or just a humble, clean piece of linen. Even a hanky.

A dressing should be highly porous. If sweat cannot evaporate through it, the skin gets moist, the dressing sodden and germs are encouraged. A dressing also helps blood clot and this encourages healing, and healing is helped by keeping the wound and the surrounding skin dry.

Dressings come in different kinds, including adhesive-backed ones, consisting of a pad of absorbent gauze or cellulose, which allow sweat to evaporate through the perforations. Pre-packed non-adhesive dressings often come with an attached roller bandage. Then there are gauze dressings, absorbent, soft and pliable, and commonly used for large wounds. These should be covered by one or more layers of cotton wool.

Bandages are not simply a means of keeping a dressing and pad in place. They do have other purposes. In first aid two kinds of bandages are used — the roller bandage, which comes in various widths from 1 inch to 4 or 5 inches wide, and the triangular bandage. To make a triangular bandage you get a square of linen or calico with each side 38 inches long. You then cut this square from corner to corner and you have two triangular bandages.

Advantage of the triangular bandage is that it can be folded to form a bandage or used open to make a sling. So it can be used to support a limb, cover a dressing almost anywhere on the body, tied on to keep splints in place, and even to exert pressure to stop bleeding.

General Rules of Bandaging. Here are some useful points regarding the application of roller bandages.

When bandaging a limb apply the bandage from within outwards and from below upwards. Always secure the first turn by a second turn or the bandage will later drop off. When you have done this secure the bandage either with a safety-pin or a strip of adhesive tape.

Apply the bandage so that each turn covers two-thirds of the previous turn. Never tie a knot over a wound or over the site of a fracture. The bandage must be tight enough to serve its purpose but not so tight that *it will injure the part or cut off the circulation of the blood. This is extremely important.* A blueish tinge of the finger or toe nail beds may be a danger signal, as is loss of sensation.

Too Tight Bandaging. Here is how you check: For an arm bandage you study the finger-nails and for a leg bandage you examine the toe-nails. Normally the nail is pink but if you press on it is goes white as the blood is pressed out of the area. When you release the pressure the nail regains its previous pink colour very quickly as the blood flows back again. If the bandage is overtight and cutting off circulation, all this changes. The pink nail looks dusky and a blueish colour and when the nail is pressed to squeeze away the blood, the blood does not flow back quickly as you release the pressure. And the nail colour stays whiteish. This is a sure sign the circulation has been stopped and you must loosen the bandage immediately and re-apply it.

BLEEDING

Bleeding may vary from trivial to severe or fatal. It can happen externally or internally. The body has certain built-in mechanisms which tend to stop bleeding spontaneously, and it is important to know this. For instance:

1. Shed blood clots, so it tends to block the damaged part.

2. The cut ends of a blood vessel will contract, so lessening the loss of blood.

3. The blood pressure drops so there is less force to push blood out of the vessel.

4. The skin vessels constrict and reduce bleeding.

Look out for the following signs and symptoms of severe loss of blood, *external or internal:*

— cold, clammy skin;

— face and lips going pale;

— casualty feels faint or dizzy;

— rapid pulse becoming weaker;

— casualty complains of thirst and is restless;

— gradually more shallow breathing, and possibly yawning and sighing;

— casualty may start gasping for air;

— casualty complains of feeling sick.

Some or all of these signs and symptoms may occur, depending on the person involved, the circumstances and the rate of bleeding.

How to Stop Bleeding

All bleeding can be controlled, sometimes even stopped by pressure. Practically every case can be checked by a firm pad and a firm bandage. If the bleeding continues it means the pad and bandage were not fixed correctly in the first place. So more pressure must be applied; this is done by putting a tighter bandage over the top of the last one, if necessary adding more dressing over the blood-soaked bandage.

If, despite every effort, you cannot stem the bleeding by direct pressure, then it may be possible to use indirect pressure — with fingers or thumbs — at the appropriate pressure point between the heart and the wound. A pressure point is where an artery can be conveniently pressed against an underlying bone to prevent the flow of blood to the wound. Such pressure may be applied while dressing, pad and bandage are being prepared for application — *not longer than 15 minutes.*

The four important pressure points are:

1. *The Carotid artery,* which runs up each side of the neck from the top of the chest wall to below the chin line.

2. *The Subclavian artery,* which runs from the chest right and left into each arm, continuing by the axillary into the armpit.

3. *The Brachial artery,* which runs along the inner side of the muscle in each upper arm (take the inside seam of a coat sleeve as a guide).

4. *The Femoral artery,* which passes into each lower limb, at a point corresponding to the centre of the fold of the groin.

Only as a last resort should you consider applying a constrictive bandage above the wound to cut off the arteries bringing blood from the heart.

Constrictive bandaging. In an emergency you can make a constrictive bandage from almost anything. A triangular bandage, a man's tie, a handkerchief, an elastic belt, a roller bandage, etc.

Tie the bandage around the limb above the wound after first protecting the skin with something soft. Tie it just tight enough to stop the bleeding. Remember, too much pressure may do harm. Having stopped the bleeding, what then?

After 15 minutes cautiously loosen the bandage and watch the wound to see if it starts to bleed again. If it doesn't, then leave the loosened constrictive bandage in position and keep a close watch on the wound. If the bleeding recurs simply re-tighten the bandage for another 15 minutes.

Get the casualty to a doctor or a hospital as quickly as possible. Attach a label indicating where you applied the constrictive bandage.

Wounds

A wound is an abnormal break in the tissue of the body which permits the escape of blood, externally or internally, and may allow germs in causing infection. There are several kinds of wounds:

1. *Clean cut or incised,* caused by a sharp instrument

like a knife or razor. They may bleed heavily.

2. *Lacerated or torn*, caused by such things as an animal's claws, machinery or barbed wire. The edges are jagged and such wounds usually bleed less than incised wounds, though dirt is more likely to be present.

3. *Bruised or contused*, caused by crushing, a blow from a hard, heavy instrument or by a fall against a hard surface.

4. *Stab or punctured*, caused by a sharp, pointed instrument such as a dagger, stiletto, needle, knife, garden fork. These wounds may look small but can be deep and dangerous.

5. *Gunshot wounds*. The entry may be small, the internal damage extensive, and the exit may be large.

Apart from bleeding, a wound carries another risk — infection. Normally, first aid means arresting bleeding, covering the wound with a sterile or clean dressing and then seeking medical help. The use of antiseptics and disinfectants on wounds is not considered part of first aid.

If the wound is over or near a joint it may be necessary to put the joint in well padded splints, or every time the joint moves it will split open the cut and never heal.

If there is also marked bleeding from the wound pressure may have to be applied alongside it or a constrictive bandage fixed above and perhaps even below the wound.

To help prevent infection in a wound which is only slightly bleeding, wash the area that is dirty from the middle outwards. Temporarily protect the wound with a sterile swab and gently clean the surrounding skin. Dry the skin with swabs of cotton wool, always wiping away from the wound.

Head wounds. The head is one area of the body where a constrictive bandage cannot be fixed. Scalp cuts tend to bleed freely and alarmingly, because blood vessels from both sides of the head mingle across the middle and a cut may have two different sets of blood vessels both bleeding simultaneously. For such cuts a large ring pad should be used to permit pressure around but *not* on the wound. A ring pad may be made by passing one end of a narrow bandage once or twice round the finger. Then bring the other end of the bandage through the loop and continue to pass it through and through until the entire bandage is used, and a firm ring made. This is applied around the wound and when bandaged presses firmly on the blood vessels coming from all sides.

Chest wounds, which suck and blow as the casualty breathes, are always serious, as they communicate with the chest cavity and air is sucked in, as the casualty breathes, instead of entering the lungs through the nostrils. Always cover such wounds immediately with a large, firm dressing and bandage — to keep the air out — and send for medical help urgently.

Internal Bleeding

An injury such as a bullet wound, a blow or a broken bone can result in internal bleeding. We can bleed into our internal cavities such as the chest, abdomen and inside the skull. We can even bleed into our soft tissues without any blood escaping through the skin or being visible to the naked eye.

Internal bleeding may remain concealed or subsequently become visible. It will stay concealed in the case of a fracture of the vault of the skull, or cerebral bleeding; bleeding into tissues associated with fractures; bleeding from the kidney, spleen or liver which have been crushed in the accident; bleeding inside the chest cavity from torn lungs.

However, even internal bleeding gives off signals which can help the first aider. You will become aware of it in the following ways:

— when blood emerges from the ears or nose, or appears as a bloodshot eye, or is swallowed and afterwards vomited, indicating a fracture of the base of the skull;
— from the lungs when blood, bright red and frothy (because it is mixed with air), is coughed up;
— from the stomach when blood is vomited. It will be bright red if vomited immediately, but if it has been in the stomach for some time it appears as either dark red, or clots, or resembling coffee grounds;
— from the upper bowel, when partly digested blood is passed in the motions, giving them a black, tarry appearance;
— from the lower bowel, when blood, looking normal, is passed in the motions;
— from the kidneys or urine, when blood escaping into the urine makes it look smokey or red.

In the case of a bruised wound, the first aider can slow up or stop bleeding by applying either a cold water compress or an ice pack. That, plus absolute rest, will ease the casualty prior to medical help.

Nose Bleeding

Severe spontaneous bleeding may result from a blow or, especially in the case of the old, perhaps be a sign of high blood pressure.

Sit the patient up and if possible put a cork or wedge between his teeth to prevent him closing his mouth. Tell him to breath through his mouth and at the same time firmly pinch the soft part of his nose. Loosen his collar and clothes around the neck. The nose may have to be held for 10 minutes before a clot forms which will seal off the bleeding. Once the bleeding does stop, the patient should rest, and not snort or fidget with his nose. If the bleeding still doesn't stop he must have medical attention.

Bleeding from The Ear

Children often tickle their ears with a hair-pin or knitting needle; adults sometimes act in this stupid way thinking they can dislodge wax. Scratching the ear with a sharp object can cause bleeding, but so can a fractured skull or disease of the ear-drum.

The ear-hole should not be plugged. Instead turn the head so that any discharge, blood, pus or serum, can come out freely, and then just cover the ear with a dry dressing to catch the blood and prevent dirt or germs getting in.

Bleeding from The Mouth

The cause may be as simple as a bitten lip during a fall. Or it could be a tongue bitten during an epileptic fit. Or the result of having a tooth removed at the dentist.

The Lip. A bleeding lip can be compressed with the fingers over a clean dressing, and then a doctor should be consulted.

A bleeding tooth socket responds best to direct pressure, through a gauze or cotton wool pad. But this must be large enough (at least one inch thick) to prevent the teeth biting through the pad. Alternatively, wrap a small cork in gauze. The patient should then be told to bite down hard for 10 to 20 minutes, supporting his chin on his hand. If bleeding continues, seek medical advice.

99

The Tongue. Again, the wound has to receive pressure. If the wound is at the front of the tongue simply grip it in gauze-covered fingers. If the wound is at the back of the tongue it is a bit trickier. Try wrapping two fingers in gauze and pressing hard on the tongue as though trying to crush it from the back towards the front teeth. In any case, seek medical aid as the wound may need stitching.

Bleeding from Palm of the Hand
Bleeding may be severe as several blood vessels are involved. Apply direct pressure and raise the arm if possible. When you find there is no fracture or irremovable foreign bodies, dress the wound and place a suitable pad over it. Bend the fingers over the pad to make a fist, then bandage the fist firmly with a folded triangular bandage, tying off across the knuckles. Support the limb in a triangular sling. When there is a fracture or irremovable foreign body present, treat the wound and support the limb in a triangular sling.

Concealed Haemorrhage
Always remember that an internal haemorrhage may be present in *any* serious accident and the moment you realise this you must direct all your efforts to getting the casualty to hospital right away — for an emergency blood transfusion and a life-saving operation.

Coughing Up Blood
This may be due to an injury. But if there has been no accident a disease of the lung, possibly tuberculosis, is likely. Such a case should be considered for rapid removal to hospital but meanwhile the patient should be nursed in a sitting position, kept quiet and still. Smoking is forbidden.

Vomiting Blood
If this is not the result of an accident, then the cause may be either a gastric or duodenal ulcer. Usually in such a case there is a long history of indigestion and discomfort after meals. The vomiting of blood comes without warning and can be fairly heavy. Again the best treatment is to get the patient to hospital immediately.

BITES

Dog Bites

Today, the threat of rabies is very real and causing tremendous concern in many West European countries. There have been one or two scares in the United Kingdom.

Rabies is almost always fatal. Death from it is painful and ugly. As yet there is no foolproof serum.

In holiday countries it is wise never to go near dogs, or other animals, in very poor areas or when it is very hot. Rabies is highly contagious.

In this country, treat a dog bite as a wound and get the casualty to a doctor, or hospital, right away, if only to confirm that it is just an innocent bite and nothing more.

Snake Bites

A snake doesn't usually attack unless you step on one or it is cornered. In Britain the poisonous viper (or adder) is the only potential killer snake. It can be found on hot dry days on heaths, commons, sandy spots, or in the woody areas of Surrey and in the New Forest.

A bite from an adder *is* dangerous. It can be fatal, unless the victim is taken to hospital immediately where he will be injected with an anti-snake serum. Initially, the victim will complain of a sharp pain. You will easily identify the bite by two puncture marks about one centimetre apart.

The trouble is, fear of being bitten often worsens the shock. Many people die from fright after a snake bite. This is what you do until medical help is available:

1. Reassure and calm the victim. Make him lie down. Don't let him get excitable and walk about.

2. Flush the wound with soapy water and wash away all venom around the wound and oozing from it. Cover with a clean cloth.

3. Support and immobilise the limb.

4. If the casualty's breathing falters or looks like stopping, start artificial respiration.

BURNS AND SCALDS

The importance of preventive measures cannot be overemphasised regarding burns and scalds, particularly where there are babies or young children. Both these injuries can be extremely serious and disfiguring. It is the extent of the area of the body affected, not so much the depth of the injury that is the danger.

Two complications most feared from such injuries are surgical shock and infection. Shock will be greater depending on the area of skin involved. If roughly a quarter to a third of the total body surface is damaged by a burn or scald then the casualty is very seriously ill, and there is a strong danger of infection. A 30 per cent burn or scald will produce a surgical shock. As a guide the head is 10 per cent of the body surface, the front of the body 18 per cent, the back 18 per cent, each arm 9 per cent. So a burn to the front of the body and both legs equals 36 per cent — well over the 30 per cent danger level. In babies and small children even a 20 per cent burn can be critical.

The area of most burns and scalds, including the clothing involved, is usually sterile initially and every effort should be made to keep it so.

There are two types of injury — the *superficial* one where the burn or scald has only damaged the outer layers of skin; the *deep* one where the entire thickness of the skin and the nerve ends are destroyed.

Burns — are caused by *dry heat*, such as red-hot metal, fire, flame, contact with hot objects like an iron, exposure to sun; *friction*, contact with a revolving wheel, wire or rope; *electricity*, an electric current, lightning; *corrosive chemicals*, such as sulphuric, nitric, hydrochloric acids, alkalis like ammonia, quicklime, caustic soda; *radiation* from X-ray overdose.

Scalds — are caused by *moist heat*, such as boiling water, steam, hot oil, tar, a poultice applied too hot.

The pain may be intense, especially with surface burns. The affected area will go red and later swell and sometimes blister, in severe cases charring. Shock becomes more intense and prolonged depending on the seriousness of the injury and the loss of fluid (plasma) and blood from the tissues.

Initially, a first aider must aim to reduce the local effects of heat, prevent infection of the affected area, relieve pain, replace fluid loss and so lessen the shock, and remove the severely injured person to hospital quickly.

Immediate treatment for the obvious hospital case would be to cover the burned or scalded area with a sterile dressing or even a very clean piece of linen.

If you have to cope without medical aid for some reason,

here is what you do:

1. To help ease the pain and diminish the heat, place the affected area gently under slowly running water or immerse in cool water, keeping it there for at least 10 minutes or until the pain eases. At this point reduction of heat is even more vital than preventing infection.

2. Remove anything like rings, belts, boots, that will constrict areas of the body bound to swell.

3. Lay the casualty down.

4. Cover the injured area with a dressing (Tulle gras squares are ideal for burns; they consist of squares of sterile gauze impregnated with a little vaseline, which means they are easily removed). The dressing can be a clean sheet, a pillow case, even a mask for the face with a hole for breathing.

5. Immobilise a badly burned limb.

6. If the casualty is conscious, give plenty of sweet drinks to help replace the fluid being lost at the injured area.

If you have either sulphonamide or antibiotic tablets in an emergency medical chest, give these in appropriate doses every four to six hours.

Do not prick blisters, breathe or cough over the burned area, or even touch it — or you increase the risk of infection.

Do not apply oil lotions or ointments.

But do reassure the casualty at all stages.

Chemical burns. You probably won't know what chemical caused the damage. So just flood the burn with running water and dilute and eliminate the chemical stuck to the surface. If you know an acid caused the burn, then neutralise with bicarbonate of soda (dissolve one or two teaspoonsful in a pint of clean water and flood it on, then apply a dressing).

If the burn was caused by a corrosive alkali like quicklime or caustic soda, first flood it with water and then make up a solution of lemon juice or vinegar diluted with an equal quantity of water, and flood this on the burn. Then apply a dressing.

If the eyes are burned get the casualty to blink his eyes under large amounts of water. But get him to hospital urgently as the burns may cause cornea scars which could permanently ruin his eyesight.

Sunburn. Even before you get that Costa del Sol suntan, while the skin is still white, you may well be a sunburn victim. Sunbathing with the body wet with sea water or sweat can also cause sunburn.

Anyone exposing the skin directly to the sun's rays risks itching, burning, redness — even superficial burns. Prevention is by very gradual exposure, as little as five minutes on the first day under a burning sun.

Best treatment is to rest in the shade, have a cold drink, and in the case of severe sunburn, seek medical aid. A dip in cool water will have a soothing effect. There are various lotions to ease slight irritation or redness of the skin.

Clothing on Fire. Immediately, see that no air can reach the victim and so fan the flames into causing further burns and greater damage. Also make sure the casualty doesn't rush misguidedly out into the open air.

If a person's clothes catch fire, first remove the heat. Quench the flames and cool the tissues with water if it is available. Otherwise, holding a blanket, rug or coat in front of you to protect yourself, approach the victim, wrap it round him, lay him flat, and smother the flames. *Never use nylon or other highly flammable, man-made material for this purpose.*

Anyone finding himself on fire when alone should roll himself over and over on the floor — smothering the flames — with the nearest heavy fabric, whether it is the curtains or the carpet.

Low Voltage Injuries. Electricity current from the domestic supply in the home — possibly a faulty connection, old wiring, worn flex to your iron — can cause a deep burn, and even stop the action of the heart and breathing.

You *must* realise that moisture and water conduct electricity. So, when the switches or wiring are faulty, and you have to try to rescue the injured person, remember you must protect yourself.

Don't touch the casualty or you may be injured by the same current which has gone through the victim's body.

Stand on some dry insulating material and with dry wood, folded newspaper or rubber, try to break the contact by switching the current off, removing the plug, or wrenching the cable free. But, again, be sure you are protected by some insulating material, and that you do not touch the casualty with your hands.

Once you have done this, give artificial respiration, if necessary, and treat burns.

CHILDBIRTH *(See Emergency Childbirth)*

CRAMP

Cramp is a sudden, painful spasm of one or a group of muscles, and it can cause momentary 'paralysis'.

Swimmers experience it when using the muscles vigorously in cold water; so do people who have sweated a lot or had acute diarrhoea and vomiting, so depriving their bodies of fluid and salt; others get cramp if they put a leg or arm into an awkward position for a time; even healthy people get it in bed; then again, it happens for no apparent reason.

If cramp follows severe loss of fluid from the body, then the casualty will need the treatment as for heat exhaustion (see page 142). Warmth and massage usually cure the trouble, but certain areas of the body will also respond if you treat cramp as follows:

In the hand — forcibly, but gently straighten out the fingers.

In the thigh — straighten the knee and raise the leg with one hand under the heel, while you press down on the knee with the other hand.

In the calf or foot — straighten the knee, and with the hand forcibly draw the foot up towards the shin *or* straighten the toes and get the casualty to stand on the ball of the foot.

In the diaphragm — this is the painful cramp called 'the stitch'. It happens to the athlete who is in poor shape for the exercise he is taking and to everybody else who is racing for that bus while the body is out of condition. Rest is the answer. Rubbing the painful area helps.

Night cramp — see your doctor, who will no doubt prescribe a nightly dose of quinine which will prevent it.

Salt deficiency. Drink lots of cold water to which has been added a half teaspoonful of salt to a pint (half a litre) of water.

CRUSH INJURIES

If someone who has been badly crushed tells you 'I am all right' after he has been rescued, don't take any notice of him. For this may happen when in fact the internal damage to the soft areas of the body is very grave.

The victim is probably very numb anyway and so cannot feel his injuries. Surgical shock may not set in right away. Often he will collapse and it is later discovered he has multiple injuries.

First aid measures, apart from sending for an ambulance, are to ensure that he can breathe properly and to stop any bleeding. Then, gently and quickly, get him to hospital.

DISLOCATIONS AND SPRAINS

You can dislocate — or displace — one or more bones at a joint, with or without it being a fracture. Joints most often displaced are those of the elbow, shoulder, thumb, fingers and lower jaw. Severe and sickening pain is one character-istic. There is usually swelling and bruising. The joint will look abnormal, even deformed, and the casualty be unable to move it.

Never treat as *just* a dislocation, give it the same support as you would a fracture. You will probably have to improvise your first aid as the limb may be displaced at an awkward angle. You must support it in that position — *don't* try and move it to the normal position. Get medical help at once.

Torn Knee Cartilage. This happens a lot in football, through a violent kick failing to connect. Also through such accidents as twisting the body while standing on one leg, slipping on a step, etc. The pain from the inner side of the knee is severe and sickening in such a case, and the knee can't usually be straightened. Any attempts to do this cause even more excruciating pain. The area over the displaced cartilage is generally very tender and because of fluid in the joint tends to swell.

Support the leg over a folded blanket and raise it. Protect with soft padding extending well above and below the joint and secure this with a firm bandage until the casualty is removed to hospital.

Sprained Joint. This is caused by the wrenching or tearing of the ligaments and tissues connected with the joint, and often accompanies a displaced cartilage. There is usually pain at the joint, swelling and later bruising. As the pain gets worse the victim is incapable of using the joint.

A good firm support is necessary. Apply pressure over the joint, which will be very tender and may often swell to a considerable size, and surround it with cotton wool pads secured by a firmly tied bandage. Or you can apply a cold compress to the joint.

In the case of a sprained ankle, if it happens out-of-doors, leave the shoe on. But support by tying a figure-of-eight bandage over it.

EMERGENCY CHILDBIRTH

Before you deliver a baby here are some guide-lines which you should follow:

1. *Send for the midwife or doctor.* In the meantime don't panic, rush around or hurry with the job you have to do. Let nature take its course.

2. *Check and prevent spread of infection.* Dirt or infection will seriously threaten the life of mother and child.

So scrub your nails and wash your hands thoroughly, if possible under running water for four minutes. Don't dry them. If they get dirty wash again. Keep your wash-basins very clean.

You and your helper should wear masks, and these are easily improvised with a handkerchief or the stronger sort of paper towel used in the kitchen.

Never let anyone help you who has a rash on the hands, a cold or sore throat.

3. *Don't pull the baby, the cord, or the afterbirth.* Let them come naturally.

4. *Don't cut or tie the cord* until the baby and afterbirth are both delivered or the cord has stopped 'beating'.

5. *Keep the baby warm.*

How do you know labour is on its way?

The prospective mother will have a 'show' of blood-stained mucus, low backache, regular contractions in the lower abdomen and, occasionally, the 'breaking of the waters'.

You must comfort and reassure her, and take her to a quiet place where she is not bothered by other people. *You* take charge until the arrival of the midwife or doctor. From now on there is plenty for you to do:

1. Prepare a cot for the baby — it may be a basket, a drawer or even a box. Get a blanket, towel or shawl to keep him warm.

2. Sterilise a pair of scissors for 10 minutes (to cut the cord).

3. If you haven't any sterile ligatures (for tying the cord) boil three pieces of 9-inch long string for 10 minutes. Or soak in methylated spirits for the same time.

4. If there isn't a bed prepare a clean surface for the mother to lie on. Protect either the bed or the surface with a sheet of plastic material or newspaper covered with a clean towel or sheet.

5. Fold a blanket into three, top to bottom, and wrap in a clean sheet — to support the top of the mother's body during the birth.

6. Have jugs of hot water ready, and either a plastic or strong bag to hold the soiled bits and pieces.

Don't fuss.

First stage. The womb contracts every 10 to 20 minutes. This stage normally lasts several hours. These contractions dilate the neck of the womb and the birth canal.

You will find the 'show' of blood-stained mucus increases, and the cramp-like pains lasting up to a minute are more frequent. As the birth progresses so they increase.

Second stage. This may start with the 'breaking of the waters' around the baby. When a pint or more of water gushes out, this means the baby is on its way.

When the mother is in the early part of this stage, keep her on her back.

When she is having the contractions she should draw her knees up, holding them with her hands, bend her head forward and hold her breath. Between contractions she should rest as much as possible.

Treatment. When a bulge appears:

1. Turn the mother onto her left side.

2. Tell her to draw her knees up, with her bottom near to the edge of the bed.

3. Support her head with a pillow.

4. Make sure her body is warm.

If she should have a bowel movement *be sure that it*

doesn't soil the birth canal. Wipe clean from in front towards the back.

The Birth

When giving birth a mother should keep her mouth open and pant in short breaths, so that the baby emerges *slowly*.

She should *not* bear down during the contractions, nor hold her breath.

The baby's head usually appears first, face downwards. But it may be bottom, foot or arm first.

Do not interfere — unless a membrane is over the face in which case it must be torn; or the cord is around the baby's neck in which case try to loop it over the shoulder or ease over the head.

Do not pull the baby or the cord — if the cord is pulled and the placenta (which becomes the afterbirth) is torn the baby may bleed to death.

Support the baby's head in the palms of your hands and wait. With the next contraction comes the baby's shoulders.

Gently but firmly grasp the baby's body under the armpits and lift *towards* the mother's abdomen.

Place the infant by the mother's legs with its head lower then the body.

Do be sure that the still-attached cord is not pulled or stretched.

A newly-born baby is wet and slippery, so remember that as you take the following action:

1. Wrap a cloth around his ankles.
2. With one finger between the ankles, grip his ankles and feet firmly.
3. Hold him head downwards.
4. Let any fluid flow from his nose and mouth by opening his mouth and holding his head slightly back.
5. Gently, with gauze or a clean cloth, remove any blood or mucus from the baby's mouth and throat.

When he starts crying put him on his side close to his mother but *not* face downwards.

If two minutes go by and he hasn't cried or shown signs of breathing, then *start resuscitation* at once — by blowing *very* gently into his lungs. *Never smack a baby into action.*

Breech delivery. If a baby appears bottom first, let well alone. Only when the shoulders emerge and the head stays inside the vagina for three minutes may a little gentle help be needed to free the baby.

Third stage. The mother will expel the afterbirth voluntarily and by contractions of her womb. She will do this best and most comfortably lying flat. So turn her on her back and separate her legs. It may be 10 minutes before the afterbirth appears. If she bleeds a lot gently massage the top of the womb (just below the navel) and it will start to do its work to expel the afterbirth.

Keep the Afterbirth — a midwife or doctor will need to check that it is all there.

The Cord. You must not do anything with the cord until the afterbirth has emerged, the cord has stopped beating and 10 minutes has gone by since the baby's birth.

Now, tie the cord very firmly in two places, one *six* inches and one *eight* inches from the baby's navel.

Unless the cord on the baby's side is secure he may bleed to death.

Cut the cord between the two ties.

Then put a sterile dressing over the cut end at the baby's navel. After 10 minutes check to make sure there is no bleeding. Then tie the cord securely *four* inches from the baby's navel.

You will need another sterile dressing for the cut end and secure it by wrapping a folded napkin or clean cloth around the baby's middle.

Don't ever use talcum powder or disinfectant on the cord or navel.

Don't ever use a dressing unless it is sterile.

It may be that the afterbirth hasn't entirely been expelled. Cover the end of the umbilical cord attached to it with a sterile dressing and tie it in place.

Care of Mother. Put a sanitary towel in position and wash the mother. Give her a hot drink and biscuits. Persuade her to sleep. Check her pulse and breathing.

Your job is done. Now you wait for the midwife and doctor.

FOREIGN BODIES
The Eye. Any injury to the eye is potentially serious.

Wounds caused by sharp tools, or even tiny bits of grit, can perforate the eyeball causing immense damage and infection, which will seriously hinder the 'working' of the eye. Blows by blunt instruments may harm the eyelids and the exposed part of the eye and also rupture the retina, the lens, and the blood vessels of the eye.

All serious eye injuries should be treated immediately by a doctor or at hospital (an eye hospital if there is one nearby). Meanwhile:

1. Stop the casualty from rubbing the eye.

2. Do *not* try to remove the foreign body if it is on the actual pupil of the eye; or embedded or stuck to the eyeball; or out of your sight but the eye is painful and inflamed.

Treat, in these cases, by closing the eyelids, covering the eye with a soft pad of cotton wool, stretching to forehead and cheek, and fixing lightly in place with a bandage. Get medical help.

3. If, when you examine the eye, you *can* see the grit or insect, and it is not on the pupil or the eyeball, treat as follows:

— site the casualty facing the light and standing in front of him, pull down the lower lid;

— take the moistened corner of a clean handkerchief and remove the offending particle;

4. If you can't see anything in the lower part of the eye

— ask the casualty to look down;

— hold the lashes of the top lid and pull them down and outwards over the lower lid. As you do so the lower lashes will sweep clean the underside of the top lid, and may dislodge the foreign body;

— if that doesn't do it, ask the casualty to blink his eye under water.

5. If you are still unsuccessful in isolating the cause of the damage, then examine the eye by folding back the top lid. Luckily there is a plate of gristle in the top lid which helps you do this. Thus:

— take a matchstick and place it against the top part of the upper eyelid and, grasping the eyelashes, fold the lid back over the matchstick.

— you may see the foreign body resting on the inside of the upper lid, and then it can be removed with the corner of a clean handkerchief.

If it is not there then study the eyeball.

— shine a small torch on the eye from the *side*, you may even need a magnifying glass to spot the mysterious object.

By the time you have done all this examining the eye will have poured with tears. The piece of grit or eyelash *should* come out with the tears. If it doesn't then it is embedded — and only a doctor or eye specialist can help. So lightly bandage the eye and get the appropriate medical help.

Chemical in the Eye. If the eye has been splashed with chemical small bits may remain in the lower lid. Wash the eye out with lots of tepid water. Or better still, if you have an eye-bath, make the casualty open his eye into that.

If you have a large enough bowl you may be able to get the casualty to plunge his face in the water and open his eye underneath the water, as if he is looking for a fish in the bottom of the bowl.

You may even be able to give a special treatment for strong acids or alkalis in the eye if you are very careful (see Injuries from Chemical Burns, page 103).

The Ear. If the object stuck in the ear is small, like an *insect*, the best thing is to float the ear with tepid water or olive oil. It should float out. Larger objects, like *beans* or *beads*, which children have a habit of inserting, should be left alone for a doctor to deal with. Though it may be possible to dislodge the object by swishing a stream of water *behind* the ear with a syringe. But do it carefully or you may damage the ear-drum.

Bleeding. If this comes from a laceration on the *outer ear*, control by the direct pressure of a dressing and bandage tied round the patient's head. If it is from the *ear canal* it may follow a head injury and a possible fracture of the skull, so a ruptured ear-drum is likely. Get medical help as quickly as possible.

Earache. This may happen at any time, and it doesn't have to be during air travel or while swimming underwater. It may be the result of inflammation from a head cold, in which case the patient should see a doctor.

In the case of earache during air travel or after underwater swimming the casualty should try to counteract the pressure by holding his nose and swallowing at the same time; *or* by blowing out his cheeks.

The Nose. Children tend to stuff beads, peas, buttons in their noses, then scream and panic when they get stuck. If the child is old enough to blow his nose, then that is all that's necessary to get rid of the object. Otherwise it is a doctor's job.

It is unwise to let a child lie down or sleep with something in the nose as it could be inhaled into the lungs. Warn a child in such a situation to breathe through the mouth until the object is removed.

The Throat. Anyone who has swallowed a fishbone or piece of gristle will remember the panic of that moment. This causes an exaggerated amount of anxiety as the victim makes frantic attempts to cough up the bone or retch. Even after a bone is removed — *always by a doctor or emergency visit to hospital* — you feel it is still there because the throat continues to hurt.

The Stomach. Again, children *do* swallow the wrong things, like coins, buttons, bits of plastic off toys, even sharp objects like pins. Smooth objects, if they're small, need not cause you too much worry. But the child should be calmed and medical help sent for right away.

Do not give the casualty anything by mouth while you wait for the doctor.

Toothache. Very painful if it persists. Dental attention is the answer. But the sufferer can help himself in the meantime by taking a pain relieving tablet or sedative, while applying warmth to the offending area. Oil of cloves soaked into a pad and clenched between the teeth is very soothing.

FRACTURES

A fracture is a broken or cracked bone. The bone may be broken and the pieces still in the correct position. Or the two pieces may have been forced out of their proper position. There may be just a crack which doesn't quite divide the bone. The bone may be smashed into many pieces. Or the bone may be partly cracked and partly bent, as sometimes happens in children — this incomplete break being known as the *greenstick fracture.*

There are many types and even a doctor won't be able to identify exactly which until the casualty has an X-ray.

So the first aider must treat the casualty as if he has a fracture, though a hospital X-ray may later show there isn't one.

Types of Fracture

Closed — this is where the bone is broken but the skin surface is intact and there is no wound.

Open — this is when the fractured ends protrude through the skin or where there is a wound, however small, leading down to the fracture.

Such a wound is especially serious because germs can enter the blood clot lying around the fracture and breed. The force of a fracture can sometimes drive the jagged ends into the brain, lungs, liver, nerves or major blood vessels. Or it can be associated with a dislocated joint. This is known as the 'complicated' fracture and, invariably, it means a surgical operation.

An alert first aider may suspect that the fracture is complicated by some other injury. For example, a case of fractured ribs will inevitably cough up blood, clearly indicating that the broken ribs have pierced the lung. This is serious, because although there is no external wound, the lungs breathe in air. And air may carry germs.

Causes of Fractures

Direct force — this is when the bone breaks at exactly where the force is applied, such as a kick on the shin, a punch on the jaw, a blow on the arm.

Indirect force — either when the bone breaks some distance from the spot where force is applied, as a fall on the outstretched hand may fracture the collar bone; or when the muscles contract violently, causing possibly a fractured knee-cap or tip of the elbow.

Signs of a Fracture

Pain — obviously the first sign, because a broken bone hurts.

Loss of power — the limb or affected area becomes inactive.

Tenderness — even from gentle pressure on the fractured area.

Swelling — there is often a lot of bleeding around a fracture and possibly extensive bruising. A swelling may

114

prevent you from recognising other signs, so when in doubt treat as a fracture.

Irregularity — where the bone lies just below the skin, such as a shin or collar-bone, you may see and feel where the line of the bone is broken. The limb may suddenly become shorter as the broken ends overlap each other, due to the contraction of the muscles. A fracture may displace another limb, as in the case of a thigh fracture, the foot flays out. Rounded bone may be noticeably and abnormally flat, as in a fractured skull.

Unnatural movement — you expect an arm or leg to move at its joints but if you notice movement at a spot where there is no joint, then there is a fracture.

Don't go out of your way to prove it by moving the casualty — if he has broken bones he will yell anyway — as you may do irreparable harm. You may increase the bleeding, damage nerve or blood vessels, or allow muscles to get between the broken bones — which, later, would considerably interfere with the broken ends knitting together.

Shock — is increased by the loss of blood. It may also be caused by either the pain or the sound and feel of the bone snapping. Or both.

Crepitus — this is the coarse, bony grating which can be heard or felt during examination of an injured part, if the ends of the bones move against each other.

Always compare an injured and uninjured limb if you can.

Treatment for Fractures

First, you stop severe bleeding and check that the casualty can breathe properly. Only after you have done this should you start treating the fracture.

It is important to treat the casualty where the accident happened, unless there is danger to your life or the casualty's. In which case carry out temporary bandaging before moving the victim to a safer place nearby.

Steady and support the injured part right away to prevent further damage, and keep this control until the fracture has been immobilised.

It is essential to keep broken bones still. This can be done by bandages or by using splints and bandages.

Never tie a bandage right over the site of a fracture. It may push the broken bones out of position. Bandages tied too tightly will cause pain and interfere with the blood flow. Soft padding before bandaging will ensure one limb doesn't chafe against another. To pass bandages underneath the casualty who is lying down use the hollows of the body, like the loins, behind the knees, the neck.

Quickest and easiest splint is often the casualty's own body. If one leg is broken, then it may be easy to tie the good leg to it, after pads have been put between the knees and ankles. In an emergency a splint can be improvised from a piece of wood, a broom handle, an umbrella, walking stick, cardboard or a firmly folded newspaper or magazine.

If splints are used they should be sufficiently rigid; they must be well padded, wide enough to fit comfortably over the limb, and long enough to immobilise the joint above and below the fracture. They can, of course, be fixed over clothing. Always tie knots over a splint or on the uninjured side. If both legs are injured, then tie the knots in front between them.

Make a check at 15 minute intervals to ensure bandages and/or splints are not fixed too firmly, as the area is likely to swell. This is particularly important when an elbow has been injured and is supported by a sling. There is always the danger, *if* dressings are too tight, of a condition called *ischaemic contracture*. This is when the blood supply is cut off. As a result the casualty may suffer life-long disability.

Special Fractures

If a person has been run over in a road accident or fallen from a great height or been badly crushed in a train then you must at once consider the possibility of a broken neck or a fractured spine.

The casualty who is conscious yet complaining of pains in the back or neck is likely to have a spine fracture. If he says he can't move his legs then you can be certain he has damaged his spine. This is a serious and grave injury. If the casualty is not handled correctly, the spinal cord may be permanently damaged and the person paralysed.

Ask the casualty to move his fingers and toes, his wrists and ankles. If he can't, he has probably lost the power in his limbs.

Touch him very gently on his limbs. Then ask him if he can feel pain or your touch. If not, there is possible loss of sensation.

If you are waiting for the doctor *do not* move him, just cover him with a blanket. But if you have to cope without medical help, place pads of soft material between the thighs, knees and ankles while someone firmly holds the casualty's shoulders and pelvis. Tie the ankles and feet together with a figure-of-eight bandage, and apply broad bandages round the thighs and knees. When it is time to move the conscious casualty carry him in the face upwards position taking care to support the head — essential where a fractured neck is suspected.

The casualty who is unconscious should be kept in a straight line like a rigid steel bar. If the spine is allowed to twist, sag or bend in *any* direction, then the spinal cord may suffer severe damage. Remember that the hollows, like the curve in the neck and in the small of the back, have to be maintained and supported. Rolled blankets and pillows will help.

This is the only time the recovery position must not be used, because of the risk of further damage to the spinal cord.

Breathing must be carefully checked and watched continuously, and mouth-to-mouth resuscitation applied if necessary. Though it must be *very* carefully done.

When the casualty is removed to a stretcher ensure that the canvas is stiffened by placing short boards of wood across it. Remember to keep the body supported by pads or alternatively pad the stretcher to support the natural curves of the neck, small of back, knees and ankles.

It is vital that the head, neck and trunk of the body are moved as if one rigid piece.

Skull fractures. Brain injury is the big risk, and can lead to very dangerous complications in a skull fracture. As a result there may be varying degrees of unconsciousness (see Unconsciousness, page 139).

Skull fractures are usually caused by a heavy blow, as when a motor cyclist is thrown from his machine. Or by a fall from a great height, when the spine shoots out of the top of the neck and fractures the base of the skull. Or when a man receives a severe smash on the lower jaw.

Signs to watch for, even after someone has regained consciousness, are blood or a corn-coloured fluid coming from the nose or ears (which may be swallowed and later

117

vomited); a bloodshot or 'black eye'; a large swelling of blood at the nape of the neck under the skin, which is a *haematoma*.

Keep an observant eye open for other injuries, such as fractures elsewhere and internal bleeding. If he is breathing normally, slightly prop up the casualty into the recovery position — that is, half way between being on his face and lying on his side. If blood or fluid is coming from his ear, place him down on that side so that it can drain out. Then lightly apply a sterile dressing.

Keep a careful check on his breathing and if it falters or stops try artificial respiration. Watch his level of consciousness and if he becomes unconscious, be sure his air passages are not blocked.

Remember, the moment a bone is broken the surrounding muscles go into a protective spasm. In the unconscious casualty this usually disappears, so you need far more care in immobilising the fracture, and ensuring splints and bandages are not too tight. For when the fracture reaction does set in those very soft parts will start to swell.

Fractured Jaw. Again there may be complications due to damage to the brain. The skull or cervical spine may also be injured.

You will have little difficulty in establishing a fractured jaw because the injured person will be in bad pain and holding his jaw to support it. Blood and saliva dribble from the mouth, the powerful jaw muscles go into spasm and the victim just makes odd noises something like an amateur ventriloquist trying to talk without moving his mouth. The teeth may be loose or even fall out, and the tongue may be bleeding badly.

Your main object will be to see that the victim is free to breathe — and ensure that the tongue hasn't fallen to the back of the throat, so obstructing the air flow.

You will need to support the lower jaw with a double loop bandage. Even a pair of women's nylon tights will do in such an emergency. Place under the jaw and tie on top of the head. This gives strong, temporary support.

Let the conscious casualty who is not severely injured sit up with his head well forward so that blood and other secretions can dribble out freely.

If there are various injuries as well as the fractured jaw

keep him in the recovery position with his head turned well to one side. Do check all the time on his breathing.

The unconscious casualty must be placed in the recovery position with the jaw well forward, chest raised and his forehead supported on a pad or on bandages. If he seems likely to vomit, turn his head to the side, supporting his jaw in the palm of your hand.

Get the patient to hospital as quickly as possible.

Fractured Ribs. This may be the direct result of a blow or a punch, as in the boxing ring, or more commonly through being crushed. This often happens when someone is moving heavy furniture in the home or is involved in a car accident.

Diagnosis is easy. The victim finds it hurts to breathe and does so in short, shallow gasps, there is sharp pain where the fracture is and, if the lungs have been punctured, blood is coughed up. There may even be a 'sucking wound' in the chest which will lead to asphyxia unless treated right away.

When the fracture is uncomplicated support the upper arm on the injured side in an arm sling. Always tie the knots on the unharmed side and place the first bandage on the lowest part of the chest. Tie when the chest is at its smallest, that is, when the casualty breathes out. The next bandage overlaps the previous one and, again, tie the knot after you have asked him to breathe out.

When the fracture is complicated immediately make airtight any 'sucking wound', which is usually the result of an open wound in the chest wall. Support the arm on the uninjured side in a triangular sling. Lay the casualty down with head and shoulders raised and the body turned slightly towards the injured side. Best way to support him is by a blanket folded lengthwise to his back. He should be taken to hospital as a stretcher case.

Fracture of the Breastbone. This fracture is rarely isolated. It usually happens with broken ribs and is the sort of thing caused by a car crash or crush injuries. It may be complicated by damage to the chest organs underneath and to the blood vessels.

Loosen the victim's clothes at the neck, chest and waist. Put him in the most comfortable position possible with his head and shoulders raised. Transport as a stretcher case on his back.

119

Fracture of the Collar-bone. Usual cause, crashing awk-wardly on the shoulder or falling on the outstretched hand. Again, it may be the result of a blow.

What is certain is, you can *see* it. Apart from pain and tenderness in the area, the arm on the injured side may hang a bit helplessly. The victim will be holding his elbow and probably bending his head towards the injured side. This relieves pain by reducing pull on the muscles. You will spot the swelling and deformity of the displaced collar-bone.

First aid is easy. Tether the arms by folding two trian-gular bandages narrow, and passing one under each arm-pit. Place a pad between the shoulder blades. Either tie the bandages together at opposite ends at the back, or secure with a third bandage. As you tighten the knots the shoulders are braced well back to correct the possible overlap of the ends of the collar-bone. Support the arm on the injured side in a triangular arm sling.

Arm Fractures. These are usually divided into fractures of the upper arm (humerus) and forearm.

If the casualty can bend his elbow then place the fore-arm of the injured limb across the chest, pointing towards the opposite shoulder. Apply a collar-and-cuff sling and then bandage the fractured upper arm to the chest for support. Do this by applying two broad bandages, one at the top of the arm just below shoulder level and the other at the lower end of the arm just above the elbow. Make sure you place some soft padding between the injured limb and the chest.

The Elbow Joint. If the fracture is near or involves the elbow joint and the elbow cannot be flexed don't try to force it. Instead, apply a long well-padded splint which stretches from near the armpit to beyond the wrist. Protect with sufficient padding between the injured arm and the body. The causalty may think he can sit or walk but he will be a lot more comfortable lying on a stretcher.

Wrist and lower end of forearm. Broken bones in both cases are usually the result of a fall on the outstretched hand. The arm/arms may be broken in about the middle of the lower part. Or the wrist may appear deformed.

First protect both the forearm and wrist by placing it on a fold of soft padding. Then support in an arm sling. Give extra strength to this support by securing the upper arm to the chest with a broad bandage fixed over the sling.

Hand and Finger Fractures. There is often a lot of bleeding into the tissues which is an added complication. Again, protect the hand by placing it on a fold of soft fabric. Support the entire arm in a triangular sling and again give extra support by bandaging the upper arm over the chest and the sling.

Leg Fractures. The same rules apply as in the treatment of the arms. If the thighbone is fractured then the best first aid is to get the casualty to hospital immediately.

Tying the knees and feet gently but firmly together with pads between the knees is a simple way of giving temporary support — before the casualty is lifted carefully onto a stretcher. The injured leg must be supported.

If medical aid isn't available, or you have to travel with the casualty a long distance over bumpy roads, then you will have to construct a well padded splint. And it will need to extend from below the armpit to the foot.

You must remember that any broken bones in the leg are serious and can cause severe shock, as well as loss of blood into the surrounding tissues. *Never underestimate a leg fracture.*

The most effective method is to use a well padded splint between the legs and the other long splint fixed to the outer side of the body and broken leg. Then firmly tie legs and splints together with bandages.

When the lower part of the leg is fractured immobilise by placing a well padded splint between the legs and then tying both legs and splint together.

Fracture of the Knee-cap. It's the sort of injury that happens to footballers, the big League boys and little schoolboys. So be prepared.

Lay the casualty on his back with head and shoulders raised and supported. Lift and support the injured leg to a comfortable position. Fix a splint along the back of the leg, reaching from the bottom to the heel. Put soft padding under the natural hollow of the ankle and secure the splint with three bandages. A figure-of-eight round ankle and foot; a broad bandage round the thigh, another round

121

the lower leg. Keep the injured leg raised and supported until the ambulance arrives.

Crushed Foot. A heavy weight usually causes these accidents. When the foot swells and the patient is in pain and unable to use his foot, then suspect a fracture.

Remove the shoe and sock or stocking very carefully, cutting if necessary. If there is a wound treat and apply a dressing. Be very gentle as there may be more than one fracture. Fix up a splint under the sole of the foot, reaching from heel to toes, and secure with a figure-of-eight bandage. Then, mainly for the casualty's comfort, place the splinted foot on its side rather than sticking up in the air.

Fracture of the Pelvis. People knocked down in traffic accidents or crushed by heavy falls of debris are the usual victims. Or those who fall heavily and awkwardly from great heights.

This sort of fracture may be complicated by injury to nearby organs, like the bladder and urinary passages, and by internal bleeding. Always treat a pelvic fracture seriously, though it may in fact be only a slight injury.

Pain in the region of the hips and loins, worsened by movement, may make the victim cry out in agony. He may describe his feelings as though his body is falling to pieces. Coughing increases the pain. He will probably be unable to stand and also want to pass water frequently, though with difficulty. If he does the urine may be darkened by blood.

The treatment is rapid transport to hospital in the most comfortable position he can find on a stretcher. But if this is delayed, you will have to secure the broken pelvis.

Make the casualty lie down on his back, knees straight. If he wants to bend his knees slightly to ease his pain support them at the back with a folded blanket. He must not pass water at this stage.

First insert padding between the legs, then tie them together. Use two broad bandages and wrap them overlapping each other round the pelvis. Tie off on the unharmed side. It is even simpler in an emergency to pass a large towel under the pelvis and secure it with two large safety pins.

FROST-BITE and HYPOTHERMIA

Mountain climbers and people living in very cold climates may get frost-bite. But it does happen to the young and old in a severe British winter.

If usually affects the extremities, the toes, fingers, nose, tips of the ears. And it is quite possible to be unaware you have frost-bite because of the very coldness of the surroundings. The frost-bitten part becomes waxy white and numb.

The person suffering from frost-bite should be taken into a house or hut where his body can warm up slowly and naturally. Don't rub the affected part, and get medical help as soon as you can.

Cold Exhaustion. Ski fanatics, mountaineers, but also those who simply are not getting enough warmth, or who have been too long exposed to the cold, can experience this insidious condition. Insidious because it can creep up on someone without them even noticing. Particularly if the victim is old and unhealthy.

You will notice, though, the cramps, the stumbling and shivering; increasing weakness of the mental and physical responses; slurred speech and difficulty in seeing; a tendency to be irritated and unreasonable; a racing pulse and 'panting' at first, yet the body still responds to the cold by shivering.

Immediately, wherever the sufferer is, protect him from the cold, wind, rain or sleet, and from wet ground under him. Wrap him in dry clothing or preferably put him in a sleeping bag. Give warm, milky drinks.

When you get the victim to base, he should have a bath and the temperature be brought up to 42°C to 45°C (107°F to 113°F). But if it was a case of prolonged exposure, he must still be given urgent medical supervision.

Hypothermia. This severe accidental cooling of the body occurs very often in babies and the elderly, who lack the strength, the ability and often the means to keep warm. Loss of heat on the outside of the body is followed by a cooling of the deep tissues and organs. Cold weather, exposure, an unheated home, lowering of resistance to cold through drink, drugs or poisoning. All these, plus possibly the added hazard of diabetes, can produce hypothermia.

Babies. They must be kept warm constantly during the first few weeks of life, as they cannot regulate their own body warmth.

The old and infirm. People living alone, especially pensioners on a poor diet, are found in a stupor or collasped outside near their homes, or even unconscious in bed. They may be fully clothed. Quite often this condition can easily be mistaken for a 'stroke' or heart attack.

The signs and symptoms are:

Babies. They are quiet and refuse food. Don't be taken in by the pink face, hands and, if you can see them, feet.

The old and infirm. They are usually in a state of collapse, very pale, the breathing slow and shallow, and the pulse barely evident.

You should aim at all costs to prevent further heat loss, to improve the body heat and circulation, and to get medical help or an ambulance. Meantime:

1. Wrap the casualty comfortably but loosely in blankets, so that the body can recover gradually.

2. If he is conscious give him tepid or warm sweet drinks.

Do not use electric blankets or hot water bottles. This is dangerous as it will cause sudden dilatation of the blood vessels near the surface of the skin, thus denying the flow of blood so badly needed for the deep tissues and internal organs. A fatal collapse may result.

POISONS

Poisons can be swallowed, inhaled into the lungs, injected through the skin by a hypodermic needle or by a snake bite, or they can be absorbed through the skin.

Poisons by mouth. These act quickly, either directly on the stomach or on the nervous system.

Stomach reaction is retching, vomiting, pain, and often diarrhoea. *Most common causes* are infected or decomposed food, poisonous berries, strong acids and alkalis, which burn the lips, mouth, gullet, and stomach, causing extreme pain.

Nervous system reaction, after poisons are absorbed into the blood, can be anything from delirium (from, say, belladonna) to fits (strychnine or prussic acid).

Poisons by inhaling. Household gas (not North Sea Gas) is the big offender, fumes from fires and stoves, car exhaust fumes, smoke; industrial gases, like carbon tetrachloride (present in some fire extinguishers and dry cleaning products); trichorethylene (found in de-greasing and dry cleaning solvents); hydrogen sulphide, cyanogen gas and cyanide fumes. All these can be very quickly fatal.

Poisons by injection. Drug addicts, particularly those on heroin, risk poisoning from the hypodermic needle. Snake venom, and bites from some animals and insects can be poisonous.

Poisons absorbed through the skin. Certain pesticides used by farmers, but also by gardeners, are the chief cause. If swallowed they can throw a person into convulsions.

Treatment: When someone is found unconscious after taking poison, the cause is seldom diagnosed at first. Anyway the casualty may be in a deep coma. The answer is to send for an ambulance and give first-aid treatment on the spot for unconsciousness. Place him so that he can breathe easily, take out his false teeth if he has them, and if breathing doesn't start begin artificial respiration. Then put him in the three-quarter recovery position so that he doesn't choke.

If the casualty is conscious and has swallowed poison recently, some of it may still be in his stomach. Ask him quickly what happened, for he may lose consciousness at any moment. If there are no signs of lip burns, which would indicate he had swallowed a corrosive, you may get the poison out of his system by making him vomit. You can induce vomiting by putting the fingers down his throat or by giving him a solution of salt water or mustard and water.

If his lips and mouth *do* show signs of burns, they will be stained yellow, grey or white. He will have a burning pain from the mouth down to the stomach, a bad breath, and cold, clammy skin. Give him water, milk or barley water to help dilute the poison and soothe him.

Of course, if the poison is swallowed some time before the discovery of the casualty, it will no longer be in the stomach, and there is little you can do.

When the casualty is removed to hospital, remember to send any particulars you know about, any remaining poison, and/or the box, bottle or container, as well as if possible a sample of the victim's vomit. All will help the doctor identify the poison.

Today, there are many substances in wide, daily use in the home that can not only be harmful but deadly.

First there are drugs, often produced as brightly coloured capsules and tablets. If left around they are an open invitation to children. Iron or anaemia tablets come into this category because they look attractive and taste sweet.

Barbiturates taken with alcohol result in many cases in collapse and death. This is a most dangerous combination of poisons.

Then there are the hair sprays and household detergents, and a hundred and one other products in cans and bottles, which may catch a child's eye and entice them to taste.

Garden plants may look pretty. But many of them are downright deadly as the name of one of them, Belladonna, or Deadly Nightshade, suggests. Laburnum pods are the sort of things children pick up — and if chewed can cause delirium and complete collapse.

On the following pages is a list of poisons, and guidance on: a) when it is safe to induce vomiting, b) whether to give an antidote to neutralise or reduce the toxicity of the poison and if so what, and c) whether to give a demulcent, a soothing drink or substance to be taken instead of or after an antidote, especially if the victim has taken a corrosive or irritant type poison.

CAPSULES, TABLETS AND MEDICINES

Poison	Induce Vomiting	Antidote	Demulcent
Amphetamines, such as slimming tablets, and 'purple hearts'	YES	NO	NO
Anti-depressants	YES	NO	NO
Anti-histamines for allergies, mosquito bites, etc.	YES	NO	NO
Atropine eye drops or travel sickness tablets	YES	Strong tea or coffee	NO
Barbiturates and sleeping tablets	YES	Strong coffee	NO

126

CAPSULES, TABLETS AND MEDICINES *continued*

Poison	Induce Vomiting	Antidote	Demulcent
Iron tablets for anaemia	YES	Bicarbonate of soda. One heaped teaspoon to a tumbler of water	NO
Digitalis heart tablets	YES	NO	NO
Tranquillisers	YES	Strong coffee	NO

HOUSEHOLD, INDUSTRIAL POISONS

Poison	Induce Vomiting	Antidote	Demulcent
Alcohol	YES	Strong coffee well sugared	NO
Ammonia	NO	Two tablespoons lemon juice *or* vinegar *or* tartaric acid solution *or* citric acid solution	YES
Anti-freeze	YES	NO	NO
Aqua Fortis (Nitric acid)	NO	Two tablespoons cream of magnesia, magnesia *or* lime water *or* one tablespoon bicarbonate of soda	YES
Benzene	NO	NO	NO
Bleaching products	YES	One heaped teaspoon sodium bicarbonate in tumbler of water	YES
Boric acid	YES	One tablespoon of magnesia	NO
Camphorated oil	YES	NO	NO
Carbolic acid	YES	One tablespoon Epsom salts *or* Glaubers salts in water *or* two tablespoons lime water	YES

Poison	Induce Vomiting	Antidote	Demulcent
Caustic Potash	NO	Two tablespoons lemon juice *or* vinegar *or* tartaric acid solution *or* citric acid solution	YES
Caustic soda	NO	Two tablespoons lemon juice *or* vinegar *or* tartaric acid solution *or* citric acid solution	YES
Disinfectants	YES	One tablespoon Epsom salts *or* Glaubers salts in water *or* two tablespoons lime water	YES
Dry cleaning fluids	YES	NO	NO
Firelighters	YES	NO	YES with heaped teaspoon bicarbonate soda
Fireworks (Phosphorus)	YES	Permanganate of Potash. A tumbler of water made up to a weak, pink solution	NEVER
Hair dye	YES	Two tablespoons of magnesia	YES
Iodine	YES	Two teaspoons starch or sodium bicarbonate in water	YES
Ink	YES	NO	YES
Insecticides	NO	Permanganate of Potash. A tumbler of water made up to a weak, pink solution	NO
Linaments	YES	One tablespoon bicarbonate of soda in a tumbler of water	NO
Liquid polish	NO	NO	YES

Poison	Induce Vomiting	Antidote	Demulcent
Methylated spirits	YES	NO	NO
Moth balls (naphthalene)	YES	NO	NO
Oil of bitter almonds (prussic acid)	YES	Half teaspoon photographic hypo in tumbler of water	NO
Oil of Vitriol (sulphuric acid)	NO	Two tablespoons cream of magnesia, magnesia *or* lime water *or* one tablespoon bicarbonate of soda	YES
Paint	YES	Half an ounce magnesium sulphate in water	YES
Paraffin	NO	NO	NO
Petrol	NO	NO	NO
Plant sprays (nicotine or arsenic)	YES	NO	YES
Rat poison	YES	Permanganate of Potash. A tumbler of water made up to a weak, pink solution	NEVER
Salts of lemon (oxalic acid)	NO	Two tablespoons cream of magnesia, magnesia *or* lime water *or* one tablespoon bicarbonate of soda	YES
Slug killer	YES	NO	YES with heaped teaspoon bicarbonate soda
Spirits of salts (hydrochloric acid)	NO	Two tablespoons cream of magnesia, magnesia *or* lime water *or* one tablespoon bicarbonate of soda	YES

HOUSEHOLD, INDUSTRIAL POISONS *continued*

Poison	Induce Vomiting	Antidote	Demulcent
Strong vinegar (acetic acid)	NO	Two tablespoons cream of magnesia, magnesia *or* lime water *or* one tablespoon bicarbonate of soda	YES
Strychnine	YES	Permanganate of Potash. A tumbler of water made up to a weak, pink solution	NO
Turpentine spirit	NO	NO	NO
Washing soda	NO	Epsom salts. One tablespoon in a tumbler of water	YES
Weed killer (arsenic)	YES	NO	YES
White spirit	NO	NO	NO

BERRIES, PLANTS AND TOADSTOOLS

Poison	Induce Vomiting	Antidote	Demulcent
Belladonna (Deadly Nightshade)	YES	Strong Coffee	NO
Black Bryony	YES	NO	YES
Cuckoo Pint (Lords and Ladies)	YES	NO	YES
Foxglove	YES	NO	YES
Henbane	YES	Strong coffee	NO
Laburnum pods	YES	NO	NO
Monkshood	YES	NO	NO
Stinking Hellebore	YES	NO	YES
Thorn Apple	YES	Strong coffee	NO
Toadstools, such as Death Cap, Fly Agaric, Panther Cap	YES	Permanganate of Potash. A tumbler of water made up to a weak, pink solution	NO

Poison	Induce Vomiting	Antidote	Demulcent
Woody Nightshade	YES	Strong coffee	NO
Yew	YES	NO	NO

RESPIRATION

Breathing, or respiration, is the process by which oxygen from the air is inhaled into the blood via the lungs. When we breathe out, carbon dioxide, a waste product, is expelled, again via the lungs.

The air we breathe comprises 20 per cent oxygen and 80 per cent nitrogen. Air enters the lungs through the nose and mouth, passing down the throat, through the voice box and into the windpipe. The top of the voice box is protected by a flap which is open for breathing but closes when food or liquid is being swallowed.

Interference with breathing prevents the body receiving its normal supply of oxygen, and this is called *asphyxia*. There are various causes which affect the airway and lungs and result in this condition:

Spasm — food, which goes down the wrong way; water, as in some cases of drowning; smoke, bronchitis, hiccups, fumes.

Obstruction — through swelling of the tissues of the throat due to injury, such as burns, scalds, stings, or swallowing corrosives; through a lot of food; through a foreign body, such as false teeth, blood, vomit; through the tongue falling to the back of the throat when a casualty is lying on his back unconscious, or in the case of a fractured jaw.

Suffocation — by plastic bags, pillows, or by being trapped in a small, airless enclosure.

Neck compression — by a tie, stocking, collar or scarf in strangulation; hanging, throttling.

Chest compression — through heavy weights, as in a mine, quarry, railway goods yard or from collapsing buildings; through being crushed against a wall or barrier or crowd, as at a football match; through damage to a lung as in a car accident, when the steering wheel smashes into the chest.

Conditions preventing the body's use of oxygen — carbon monoxide poisoning, by car exhaust fumes or household gas (not North Sea natural gas); prussic acid gas, which prevents the tissues from using the oxygen present in the blood; air lacking oxygen, such as in tunnels, disused shafts, smoke-filled buildings; change in atmospheric pressure, like high altitudes and deep-sea diving; continuous fits, preventing regular breathing.

Depression of the brain and nerves which control breathing — through the paralysing effect of electric shock and lightning; through poisons such as morphine, which acts directly on the brain, barbiturates, industrial gases, pesticides; through muscle contraction as in lockjaw; through paralysis, as in polio, apoplexy, or injury to the spinal cord.

Look out for the following signs and symptoms of asphyxia:

Breathing — in the early stages there is shortness of breath, and increasing difficulty leading to gasping with frothing at the mouth.

Pulse — becomes rapid and marked swelling of the neck veins will be apparent.

Congestion — the head and neck, face, lips, eyelids and nail beds of fingers and toes may become a dusky blue. In carbon monoxide poisoning there is no cyanosis of the face because carbon monoxide makes the blood a pink colour. So the face and lips look a healthy pink instead of the more usual congested blue/purple colour.

As the asphyxia worsens the casualty starts to lose consciousness. The embarrassed heart beats slowly and irregularly, breathing becomes intermittent and then stops. The coma deepens until the heart stops beating and the casualty dies.

Treatment of Asphyxia. The vital need is to eliminate the cause, if possible, ensuring that the air passages to the lungs are open and oxygen is reaching the blood. And to apply artificial respiration. This can be continued in an ambulance or lorry while the casualty is being rushed to hospital for other means of resuscitation.

Make no mistake, speed, the immediate application of artificial respiration is what saves lives.

Artificial Respiration

There are several methods of artificial respiration. The

most effective is that heavily favoured by the experts — mouth-to-mouth (mouth-to-nose) resuscitation.

There is one snag about the mouth-to-mouth method. The casualty may also have facial injuries which make this impractical, or poison on the lips, or skin which might be a danger to a first aider. Then you would have to adopt the second best choice, the Silvester Method.

Mouth-to-mouth Respiration. Secret of the success of the mouth-to-mouth method is that you can start it *immediately* — wherever you find the casualty and with little or no preparation.

Because of the force of the pressure you make you can force air past any minor obstruction, such as fluid in the nostrils as in drowning. Some of it will be forced up and out. You don't have to delay and up-end the casualty, and try to drain out water before you start. But if you find you can't get air into his lungs, turn the victim on his side, thump his back to dislodge any foreign matter from the back of his throat, and clear his mouth.

It is vital to check that the tongue hasn't fallen to the back of the throat. If someone is unconscious and on his back this often happens and will obstruct the air passage.

But, if you tilt his head fully backwards and push his jaw forwards and upwards towards the sky above him, his tongue will be pushed out of the way into its correct position.

If the victim is capable of breathing this may be all that is necessary; he will gasp and start to breathe. Place him, then, in the recovery position.

If the casualty is not breathing, maintain that grasp — his head tilted backwards and the jaw jutting skywards as you support the nape of his neck.

Having ensured that air can reach the victim, loosen his clothes at the neck and waist.

Now, still maintaining that grasp, take a deep double breath yourself and place your mouth in an airtight fit over the casualty's mouth. Then you force *your* breath into *his* lungs quickly and strongly three or four times, to saturate the blood with oxygen.

Pinch his nostrils together with your fingers. Then, once every six seconds blow into his lungs until the chest rises. Remove your mouth and watch the chest fall. Repeat and continue inflations at your natural rate of breathing.

Alternatively, seal off the casualty's mouth by closing his lips, and, mouth-to-nose, blow in through his nostrils.

With children in distress take extra precautions. Seal your lips round the child's mouth and nose and blow *gently* with shallow puffs of air into his lungs. When the chest rises remove your mouth and as the chest falls, repeat the inflations. Do this rather more quickly, once every three seconds.

If the heart is beating normally, continue artificial respiration until natural breathing is restored. Then send for the ambulance after placing him in the recovery position.

If the heart is NOT beating you will know because the victim's colour will be blue/grey, the pupils if visible widely dilated, and the pulse in the neck not registering, so put him on his back on the floor and strike his chest smartly on the lower part of the breastbone with the edge of the hand. This may re-start the heart beating. If there is still no response start external heart compression immediately.

Remember: in respiratory arrest it is safe and sensible to start artificial respiration while breathing appears to be failing.

In *cardiac (heart) arrest* external heart compression should not be begun unless you are sure the heart has stopped beating.

External heart compression. Kneel at the side of the victim and feel for the lower half of the breastbone. Place the heel of your hand on this part of the bone, keeping the palm and fingers off the chest. Cover this hand with the heel of the other hand. Then, with arms straight, rock forwards pressing down on the lower half of the breastbone (this can be done for about 1½ inches in an unconscious adult).

The pressure should always be firm and controlled, not erratic or harsh — otherwise there may be risk of damage to the ribs or internal organs.

In adults, repeat the pressure at least 60 times a minute.

In children, try light pressure with one hand but at about 80 to 90 times a minute. *In children under 10*, try very light fingered pressure at about 100 times a minute.

You will soon see how effective your first aid is — by the return of the casualty's colour; by the pupils of the eyes becoming smaller; by the feel of the carotid pulse in the neck.

Keep going until the ambulance arrives, and you may need to keep up resuscitation until the casualty reaches hospital.

The Silvester Method. If you cannot give mouth-to-mouth, or mouth-to-nose resuscitation to revive someone — perhaps because of facial injuries — the Silvester Method is the best alternative. What is more, it also allows you to use external heart compression (as described above) when necessary. This then is the Silvester treatment:

1. Clear the air passages of any obstruction that can be reached with the fingers, by tilting the casualty's head back. Check the mouth in the same way.

2. Lay the casualty on his back on a firm surface and raise his shoulders on a folded jacket or on something else, and allow his head to fall back.

3. Kneel astride the casualty's head, facing towards his feet, and grasp his arms at the wrists.

4. Cross his arms and press them firmly over the lower part of his chest. This forces air *out* of the lungs.

5. Rock your body forwards and press down on the casualty's chest over his crossed arms.

6. Release the pressure and with a sweeping movement draw the casualty's arms backwards and outwards above his head, pulling his arms towards the ground. This movement should cause air *to enter* the lungs.

7. Repeat these movements rhythmically about 12 times a minute in an adult, taking two seconds for the chest pressure movement, and three seconds for the arm lift.

When a casualty is on his back there is always the danger that he may inhale vomit, mucus or blood. You can reduce this risk by turning his head to one side and a little lower than the rest of his body.

If there is no improvement in the casualty's colour, turn him on his side and strike him sharply on the back between his shoulder blades. This will clear any obstruction. Then continue artificial respiration until either the casualty starts to breathe normally, or a doctor decides further effort is pointless.

RUPTURE

This is a swelling, sometimes known as an abdominal hernia, which pops through a weak spot in the abdominal wall. It happens in the groin, the navel, through the scar of an abdominal operation; even intestines rupture.

Anyone over-exerting themselves in sport or exercises, lifting heavy objects, coughing or even when straining on the lavatory through constipation, can cause a rupture. The swelling may appear suddenly after a period of heavy work. Or it may come on gradually over the months, getting larger and larger.

Faced with such a swelling, the question is — is it an enlarged gland or a rupture? The diagnosis can be settled by asking the victim to cough. If with every cough the swelling enlarges, or if you can feel an impulse in the swelling during coughing, then it *is* a rupture.

Sometimes a man or woman goes around with this condition, quite happily living with it. But there comes a time when it becomes *irreducible*.

A ruptured intestine may cause an obstruction and with it severe pain and distress. The area is especially tender, and the sufferer may vomit at times. This is what happens when someone has a 'strangulated hernia'. These signs and symptoms should tell you it is an immediate surgical problem.

Most effective treatment for someone experiencing severe discomfort or bad pain with a hernia is to reassure him, and make him lie down. Support the head and shoulders, bend and support his knees. If he vomits or seems likely to, place him in the recovery position. Call the doctor.

SHOCK

Shock is a condition resulting from loss of blood or some terrific *emotional* upset to the nervous system. It results in a lessening of the vital functions of the body arising from lack of blood supply. Someone suffering from shock will convey the following signs and symptoms:

— his skin will become extremely pale, go cold and clammy, and there will be profuse sweating;
— he may feel faint or giddy or have blurred vision;
— he may feel sick and may vomit;
— he may be very anxious;
— he may complain of thirst;
— his consciousness may be clouded;

— his pulse quickens, then tends to become weak and thready;

— his breathing is shallow and rapid.

Emotional Shock. A really bad fright, like seeing your child scalded, your husband knocked down, or hearing of the death of a loved one, often results in emotional shock. Your eyes or senses register the disaster and send a message to the brain; the brain, appalled by what has happened, is stricken with a nervous paralysis. This, in turn, causes anaemia of the brain and drop in blood pressure, which affects the higher nerve centres. As a result, the person may faint and then recover.

No blood has been lost so no treatment is necessary. Simply keep the patient in a horizontal position or raise the lower part of the body so that the head is lower.

A word or warning. Someone suffering from emotional shock may come round moaning and weeping, or even be violently hysterical. She or he will need kindness and sympathy, or even gently restraining. Don't leave the patient unless you are sure recovery is complete.

Surgical Shock. The body holds a total of 10 or 12 pints of blood. We can lose one or two pints without undue harm — after all blood donors can give this quantity. But, if we lose more, then the centres in the brain become anaemic and surgical shock sets in.

Anything which greatly reduces the volume of blood circulating to the brain produces surgical shock. It can be a massive haemorrhage from a wound, a large concealed haemorrhage into one of the body's cavities, a severe crash injury or extensive burns or scalds.

The obvious and vital treatment is an urgent blood transfusion to restore the body's blood quota. Nothing must stand in the way of getting this transfusion to the patient as fast as possible, otherwise there will be irreversible damage to the brain from which it cannot recover.

First aid treatment for surgical shock:

1. If there is severe bleeding, stop it.

2. See that there is no interference with breathing, especially during the journey to hospital.

3. If there is a sucking wound of the chest cover it with a large dressing to cover the hole.

4. The patient will probably be having an operation and therefore an anaesthetic. So do not give any drinks. An empty stomach is necessary for an operation.

5. With a fractured limb do the minimum necessary to immobilise it for transport.

6. Cover the casualty with a single blanket. Don't try to warm him up even if he seems to be shivering.

7. Don't give the patient cigarettes in mistaken sympathy.

8. If there is no head, chest or abdominal injury, raise the foot of the stretcher so the casualty is kept in the head low position.

While working fast keep calm in front of the patient to reassure him. Do all the major essentials to save life and quickly remove him to hospital.

STINGS — Bee, Wasp and Hornet

Stings from bees and wasps in Britain also cause a local tissue reaction and poisoning.

If the sting is in the mouth there may be a dangerous swelling which can obstruct breathing. This needs urgent medical attention and you must tell the doctor what has happened so that he can bring an adrenalin injection with him. Multiple stings also need immediate medical attention. Meanwhile give the victim a mouthwash of one teaspoonful of bicarbonate of soda in a tumbler of water. If the condition gets worse, place in the recovery position and give him ice to suck.

A bee sting is peculiar in that it has a barb shaped like an anchor and the bee cannot retract it. So the victim not only has a painful sting, and its complications, but the whole of the bee's stinging apparatus still embedded in the skin. This must be removed without squeezing the sting bag or more poison will be injected. Ease out with the point of a sterilised needle and wipe off with a clean handkerchief.

Afterwards, apply an anti-histamine cream or calamine lotion. Or even surgical spirit or a weak ammonia solution or a solution of bicarbonate of soda.

STRAINS

While a *sprain* means a joint has been wrenched or the joint ligaments torn, a *strain* is an injury to the muscle.

Violent or unexpected exercise may tear a few muscle

fibres and then the whole muscle goes into a protective spasm — causing severe cramp and swelling. The pain is swift and sharp.

All you can do is treat as a fracture, steadying and supporting the injured part, and get the victim to hospital for X-ray.

UNCONSCIOUSNESS

This condition is due to interruption of the brain's normal activity through interference with the functions of the nervous system and circulation.

If a person is only partly conscious he is in a *stupor* and if he is completely unconscious he is in a *coma.* You can establish exactly which by shouting a question at the casualty. If he answers you are getting through to him so he is in a *stupor.* Unless of course he is normally deaf. No response may mean he is in a *coma, faking,* in a *hysterical state,* or *dead.* A first aider should never presume death, that is a doctor's job.

If you pull back the casualty's eyelids and they flutter or resist, he is in a stupor; when he doesn't respond it shows the muscles are not working and he is in a coma. You can also deduce the condition by retracting the eyelids and shining a torch into the casualty's eyes. The pupils will contract if he is in stupor, and dilate when the light goes off. In coma the pupils will not move if a light is shone directly into the eyes. A person in a deep coma will have widely dilated pupils as well as being unresponsive to light.

A casualty under the effects of morphia or other drugs will have pin point pupils, which is one clue that the casualty has possibly taken an overdose.

Causes of Unconsciousness

Apart from asphyxia (lack of oxygen reaching the blood) and shock, the next most common cause of unconsciousness is a head injury. Others are, a stroke, poisoning, heart attacks, epilepsy, convulsions in young children, diabetic emergencies.

A head injury, such as a blow on the skull, may so rock the brain inside that the casualty becomes either dazed or unconscious. This is called *concussion.* It may last a few minutes or several days. The first sign of recovery is often an attack of vomiting. When he regains consciousness the casualty may suffer from loss of memory and be unable to remember what hit him or how he came to be in hospital.

If the only damage to the brain is concussion and a shaking-up then the casualty gradually recovers. But sometimes there is more severe damage. There may have been bleeding into the skull or laceration of the brain. The blood collects and compresses on the brain and this condition is *cerebral compression*.

Concussion may pass into compression without the casualty regaining consciousness. Sometimes the casualty comes round from the concussion then slips into a coma from late development of compression. A concussion case is quiet and just appears to be deeply asleep, but when compression sets in the whole picture changes. He becomes red-faced with a slow bounding pulse, deeply unconscious, and with noisy breathing; there may even be twitching of the limbs or even convulsions. The pupils of the eyes may be unequal or widely dilated and not react to light.

A man suffering with high blood pressure may suddenly have a stroke. Either a blood vessel bursts in the brain (a cerebral haemorrhage) or a blood vessel clots up (cerebral thrombosis). The absence of any suggestion of an accident gives a clue. Never be caught out by assuming an unconscious man is drunk, just because his breath smells of alcohol.

First Aid for the Unconscious

The aim is to ensure there is no obstruction to breathing, and also to get urgent medical attention for the casualty.

1. (a)   Make sure the air passages are not obstructed; remove false teeth and put in a safe place; clear the mouth of mucus, blood, vomit and any detached teeth, using a handkerchief when necessary.

(b)   Ensure there is plenty of fresh air to breathe, open windows and doors, or remove casualty from harmful gases or contaminated atmosphere.

2. Slightly raise his shoulders and turn his head to one side in case he vomits.

3. If breathing begins to fail or stop, immediately start artificial respiration. If the breathing is noisy and sounds as though water is bubbling in his chest, move him into the three-quarter prone position.

4. Cover him with a blanket and place one under him if possible. But don't warm him up with hot water bottles.

5. If removal to the hospital is delayed check the casualty's responses and pulse rate at intervals, and keep a written record for the doctor.

6. If the casualty regains consciousness, talk to him reassuringly, moisten his lips with water. If he is restless prevent him from harming himself.

Do not give him a drink.

Do not leave him unattended.

Special Causes of Unconsciousness

Epilepsy. This condition can happen at any age but usually first appears in young people. People suffering with epilepsy are liable to recurrent attacks — and they may be minor or major.

In the case of a minor attack the individual becomes pale and the eyes fixed and staring. He is not conscious of his surroundings. The attack may be similar to a faint — and should be treated like one — with the victim soon resuming normal activity.

A major attack is a true epileptic fit. Often the victim has a premonition that he is going to have a fit, for he feels strange, irritable, restless, and in a dreamy state.

The fit consists of four stages:

1. The victim suddenly falls to the ground, cries out, and then lapses into unconsciousness.

2. He remains rigid for a few seconds, and his face and neck become congested.

3. All the muscles start to jerk in a series of alternate contraction and relaxation. These are the convulsive spasms. Breathing through the clenched jaw is noisy; froth may sometimes come from the mouth, possibly blood-stained if the tongue is bitten. During the attack the victim may lose control of the bladder and bowels, and pass urine and motions involuntarily.

4. The jerking gradually passes off and later a very sleepy person comes to and looks surprised to see you. Though he may be confused, with loss of memory of recent events and need a little while to gather himself together. He may even wander about without realising what he is doing, then exhausted, fall into a deep sleep.

Aim of the treatment is to prevent the victim from harming himself and to keep his air passages clear. Try to get something like a knotted handkerchief between his teeth on which he can bite without hurting the tongue. If the tongue is bleeding freely then turn the victim into the three-quarter prone position so that the blood can run out of the mouth and not down his throat and choke him. Apply the general treatment for unconsciousness and, as soon as the attack has passed off, seek medical aid for the fit and for the tongue if bleeding has occurred.

Heatstroke. Tennis players on the world's professional circuits, footballers playing in hot weather, men working in a foundry or below decks in a ship's stokehole, will sweat many pints of fluid in a day. And with the sweat goes much of the body's salt. Newcomers to a very hot climate, especially humid heat, may suffer from the excessive heat. This is often aggravated further by gastro-intestinal upsets with vomiting and diarrhoea. The result is:

Heat Exhaustion. The symptoms may be any or all of the following: cramp, headache, vertigo, vomiting or collaspe and unconsciousness.

The first aid for heat exhaustion is to keep the casualty cool and rapidly replace the fluid and salt lost by giving lots of drinks of salt and water. One quarter of a teaspoonful of salt to a tumbler of water, and flavoured with some fruit cordial, is best.

If the casualty has sweated until he can sweat no more or is one of those people who cannot sweat enough anyway — high humidity, lack of air, malaria or other debilitating illness may bring it on — then heat exhaustion becomes:

Heat Stroke. Symptoms are more sudden. The temperature is likely to be at least 40°C (104°F), and the victim restless (if conscious), complaining of a headache, dizziness and feeling hot. The face is flushed, the skin dry to touch, the pulse full and bounding; a stupor or even a coma may result.

The chief object is to reduce the person's temperature as fast as possible, though not so suddenly as to cause shock as well. Place him in a cool spot and wrap him in a wet, cold sheet, and if possible put an ice-bag to the head.

Keep a check on the body temperature and when it has dropped to around 101 degrees, wrap him in a dry sheet but let him stay in a cool place where there is a draught.

If the temperature soars again, repeat the wet treatment. As soon as the victim is conscious treat him as for heat exhaustion or, if his condition doesn't improve, get him to hospital.

Diabetic Coma. People suffering from diabetes (a result of the pancreas producing insufficient insulin to keep the blood sugar at a normal level) are liable to two types of coma. One from the disease, the other from too much insulin.

Insulin or other drugs are prescribed for a diabetic to maintain the sugar level in the blood. But there is then the danger that the diabetic may have more insulin that he needs, because he has already used up the sugar through excessive exercise; or he may not have eaten enough; or he may have accidentially given himself too much insulin.

Insulin Coma. The diabetic is pale, sweating a lot, his pulse is racing, his breathing shallow but his breath clean; his limbs may be trembling, he may appear to be aggressive or drunk; he may faint or become unconscious quite quickly.

Diabetic Coma. The diabetic's skin is dry, his face flushed, his breathing deep and sighing and his breath smells strongly of acetone (like nail varnish or musty apples). He gradually sinks into a diabetic coma.

There may be uncertainty as to whether the person is suffering from too much or too little insulin. First of all, search the sufferer for a card showing that he is a diabetic, and for lumps of sugar which someone on insulin often carries. Look for marks of recent injections in the arm, thigh or abdomen. Waste no time in getting medical aid and, in the case of a diabetic coma, get the sufferer straight to hospital. Treatment in the meantime should be as follows:

If conscious — (the victim can confirm he is a diabetic), don't hesitate, give him a drink sweetened with two full tablespoons of sugar, or lumps of sugar or other sweet products. The patient who improves quickly has obviously had too much insulin. But ensure he gets more sugar in case he relapses into a coma.

If unconscious — place in the recovery position and arrange for immediate admission to hospital.

Fainting. This results directly from a temporary inadequate supply of blood to the brain.

A fright, horrifying incident, bad news, pain, fatigue, even long periods sitting or standing in a hot, stuffy place —

all can cause fainting. It may begin with a gradual feeling of faintness, or there may be a sudden collaspse. The casualty usually goes deathly white, even greenish white in colour, yawns, sways and feels unsteady, with beads of sweat on his face, neck and hands as his consciousness clouds.

Treatment is twofold. If he is about to faint, reassure him and urge him to breathe deeply and flex his muscles to help the blood circulate. Loosen his clothes. Sit him down and thrust his head well down between his knees and when he feels better, let him sip a cold drink. Take him to a cool spot where there is plenty of fresh air.

Remember, the faint may be a prelude in some people to an hysterical attack.

If the faint is complete — the person's face pale, his skin cold and clammy, his breathing shallow and his pulse weak and slow at first, but gradually increasing in rate — then you are dealing with someone who is unconscious.

Lay the casualty down with his head turned to one side. Raise the legs slightly above the level of his head and loosen the clothes at the neck, chest and waist. Place him in the recovery position if his breathing is difficult — and wait. He will recover. Now is the time to reassure him and raise him into a sitting position, giving him sips of water if he wishes.

You can tell when someone who has fainted is recovering, because the colour returns to the skin. If recovery is slow and not complete, then hospital treatment will be necessary.

Heart Attacks. There are four kinds of heart attacks. The two most acute are *Coronary Thrombosis* (obstruction of a coronary artery in the wall of the heart) and *Angina Pectoris* (severe pain in the chest). Most rare are called *Stokes Adams attacks* (slow heart beat). Finally there is *Heart Failure* (tired heart that can't cope).

Coronary Thrombosis. The victim is suddenly gripped by an excruciating vice-like pain in the centre of the chest. It is severe and continuous and the pain may extend into the neck and down each arm. Sometimes it is mistaken for indigestion.

The victim usually looks shocked and feels it. The severe pain will stop him from what he is doing. He may feel giddy and collapse.

This is all due to a clot forming in one of the arteries

that gives the heart muscle its blood supply. Remember, it is vital that the victim doesn't move — movement may be the last straw that stops the heart.

Send for the ambulance immediately, and meantime very gently ease the victim into a comfortable position with his head and shoulders raised on two or more pillows, or support him in a sitting position, if this eases his breathing. Artificial respiration or external heart compression may be necessary while you wait, and even en route to the hospital.

Not all cases develop a clot of blood, some just develop a spasm of the artery. This is called:

Angina Pectoris. Excitement or over-exertion brings on an attack of pain in the chest. The channels of the arteries supplying blood to the heart have become too narrow for an adequate supply to the heart muscle when it is working harder 'than normal. The pain often spreads to the left shoulder and arm and to the fingers, even to the throat and jaws.

The victim won't be unconscious, simply standing or sitting clutching his chest complaining of pain and probably trying to find the trinitrin tablets prescribed by his doctor for just such an emergency, or trying to break and sniff one of the glass capsules angina sufferers often carry on them. If he has such treatment on him, give it to him, and keep him still and quiet in the same way as a coronary victim. Again, send for medical aid.

Stokes Adams attacks. In these the heart beats so slowly that there is not enough blood going to the brain and the person literally faints.

First aid treatment is similar to that given in an ordinary faint. Lay him down and send for medical help. The pulse may be as slow as 10 beats to the minute. Any relatives present will no doubt know about his liability to such attacks.

Heart Failure. Chronic heart disease, high blood pressure, or severe chest disease sooner or later place such a heavy burden on the heart that eventually it just gives up. The victim is blue-lipped and breathless and may not even be able to speak, just gasp. Keep him still in a sitting position and send for medical aid.

INDEX